Management of Childhood Obesity

Elizabeth Poskitt has practised and taught paediatrics in the UK and overseas. Her experience includes over 20 years running clinics for obese children, first in Birmingham and then Liverpool. She is co-founder of the European Childhood Obesity Group. She was awarded an OBE in 1998.

Laurel Edmunds has worked with children and their families for over 16 years and has researched childhood obesity issues for the past 14 years, including two years in practice. She was one of five Specialist Advisors to the House of Commons Health Committee's enquiry into obesity and was a Co-opted Expert for the NICE Guidelines.

Management of Childhood Obesity

Elizabeth Poskitt

and

Laurel Edmunds

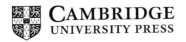
CAMBRIDGE
UNIVERSITY PRESS

CAMBRIDGE UNIVERSITY PRESS
Cambridge, New York, Melbourne, Madrid, Cape Town, Singapore, São Paulo, Delhi

Cambridge University Press
The Edinburgh Building, Cambridge CB2 8RU, UK

Published in the United States of America by Cambridge University Press, New York

www.cambridge.org
Information on this title: www.cambridge.org/9780521609777

First published 2008

Printed in the United Kingdom at the University Press, Cambridge

A catalogue record for this publication is available from the British Library

ISBN 978-0-521-60977-7 paperback

Contents

Foreword

Childhood obesity is one of the most serious problems facing the developed world. It is damaging to the medical and psychological well-being of our children, and casts a shadow on their future health as adults, leading to serious illness and ultimately premature death.

This book, written by world-renowned leaders in the field, should be used as a practical tool in the management of the overweight child rather than left on the shelf to gather dust like some medical books. Its pages should become well-thumbed by front-line health care professionals, commissioners and policy-makers alike. It would even be acceptable to turn back the corners of the pages, and use light pencil markings on the margin to highlight important passages, because unlike many volumes, this represents first-hand experiences of practical childhood obesity management, combined with a profound scientific, clinical and social appreciation of the condition and its ramifications.

Weight management in children is one of the most difficult challenges faced by health care professionals who cannot change the environment which leads to the weight problems in the first place. Only the government, food, retail, advertising industry, schools, planners and other authorities can do that. Sweets and chocolates still appear at supermarket check-outs, fast food outlets still sell vast portions of cheap, unhealthy food at all times of day and night on every street corner. Many schools still provide inappropriate meals and too little physical activity for their students; many food and drink companies still use sports and entertainment idols to flog their wares, thereby putting enormous pressure on children to obey what is already a powerful instinct to eat more and more. Whilst we are waiting for the environment to change, primary and secondary care workers have the job of managing the childhood obesity epidemic in our clinics, one person, and one family at a time.

As a general practitioner, I encounter childhood obesity every day, and it is one of the most difficult challenges I face. However, a successful result and a healthy and happy child are the most rewarding and satisfying outcomes for the primary care team and for the family. As well as providing the scientific and academic background to childhood weight issues, the authors share their immense practical experience of what actually works in the management of the overweight child in a sympathetic and practical way, and for this reason, the book should be required reading for everyone involved with childhood weight problems.

David W. Haslam, MB BS

General Practice Principal

Clinical Director National Obesity Forum

Preface

When one of us first started working with overweight and obese children in the early 1970s the admission that she ran an obesity clinic for children was greeted with wry amusement or the comment 'You don't achieve anything do you?' Today the prevalence of childhood overweight and obesity in not only the UK but most westernized societies and increasingly in less affluent countries too has changed this attitude. The comment is now not whether we achieve anything but an imperative that we must achieve something if we are to prevent the present generation of young people having lifetimes of high morbidity and mortality as consequences of their excessive fatness. Yet, for all the concern about obesity, there is no 'magic bullet', 'wonder diet' nor consensus view on how to manage the condition. This book does not pretend to answer that dilemma but to present guidance which we hope will support those trying to help these children.

Throughout the book we use both overweight and obesity, often together, to describe children who are likely to have significant increases in percentage of body weight as fat. The mixed terminology relates to the fact that most children are diagnosed as 'obese' because they have a high body weight and thus an abnormal relationship between weight and height for age (whatever method is used). Technologies that have been developed to be more specific about body composition in most cases do not directly measure fat in the body (see Chapter 2). Estimates of body fat are largely confined to research studies. Thus we prefer to use overweight as a descriptive term for the presumed overfat children in whom we are concerned. The difference in the definitions of overweight and obese in practical terms is usually one of degree and has little significance for pathology except that the more severely affected – the obese – are generally more prone to the problems associated with being overfat. However we do recognize that there are problems with the clinical definition of overweight in that it can include children who have excess lean, rather than fat, tissue. In our modern, relatively inactive, society such children are distinguishable in most cases by their obvious athleticism or their extreme height for age. A further reason for not confining ourselves to the term 'obese' routinely is that some see this as a derogatory term. We have no wish to diminish further the self-esteem of a group in the population who may already have a poor image of themselves and feelings of ostracization and who can justifiably argue that they deserve the respect that should be given to all.

The overweight/obese children who are the subjects of this book are those presenting in the community, in primary care or at a general paediatric clinic. Our advice is therefore aimed at health care practitioners (HCP) in the community. Perhaps we can also provide some help for those working in general paediatrics and, at the other end of the scale, for parents making their own efforts to cope with children whose rapid weight gains and increasing fatness are concerning. With obesity such a highly prevalent problem, the majority of those who need to control their weight will probably never get beyond advice at the primary care level. For this reason we deal no more than briefly with investigations and therapies likely to apply only to the relatively few obese children who receive hospital specialist care. However we see it as important to recognize and distinguish those overweight/obese children who do need detailed investigation or very specific, possibly invasive, management.

Modern medical management is perceived as needing an evidence base. The gold standard for evaluating management is the double-blind randomized controlled trial. The advice for the management of child obesity has a limited evidence base which has been extensively reviewed in the process of developing the UK National Institute of Health and Clinical Excellence (NICE) Guidelines on the management of obesity (NICE 2006). With such a multifaceted condition as obesity and with the variety of diets, activities, lifestyles and psychosocial considerations which contribute to the condition at the individual level, it may be impossible – at least in a free society – to put some aspects of management to the test. However overweight/obese children cannot be allowed to get progressively fatter just because there is no absolutely proven method of management. We have tried to follow those NICE (2006) Guidelines relevant to the children, families and communities we aim to reach. In addition we incorporate what we believe common sense and our experience in practice and research indicate as reasonable recommendations to support that management which already has an evidence base.

The expansion of research into childhood obesity which has taken place in recent years is a very positive development. A mass of evidence is being gathered and gradually being published – as the NICE (2006) Guidelines show. Research programmes developing effective management for childhood overweight/obesity do not always transfer easily into practices that are clinically and financially sustainable. There is still a long way to go before the obesity epidemic in children is under control. It is therefore important that all involved do all they can to reduce the effects of the epidemic on physical and psychosocial health. It is time to achieve change: something must be done. We make suggestions for what this 'something' might be.

Acknowledgements

We are obviously indebted to the overweight and other children and their families who have provided us with clinical experience and opportunities for research over many years and without whom our comments would have no rational basis. However, in the immediate circumstances, our particular gratitude is to David W. Haslam of the National Obesity Forum who has taken time to read the book and give us his comments as well as providing a Foreword and to Louise Diss of TOAST (The Obesity Awareness and Solutions Trust) for likewise looking through the book and giving us her advice. As sole authors the responsibility for statements made in the book is ours alone.

Abbreviations

ALSPAC	Avon Longitudinal Study of Parents and Children
AR	adiposity rebound
%BF	percentage body fat
BI	bioelectrical impedance
BMI	body mass index
BMR	basal metabolic rate
BP	blood pressure
CDC	Center for Disease Control (USA)
CMO	Chief Medical Officer
CT	computerized tomography
DEXA	dual X-ray absorptiometry
DH	Department of Health
FFQ	food frequency questionnaire
FSA	Food Standards Agency
GDA	Guideline Daily Amount
GI	glycaemic index
GP	general practitioner
HCP	health care professional
HDL	high density lipoprotein
HFSS	high fat, high sugar, high salt
ICP	intracranial pressure
IOTF	International Obesity Task Force
ISC	Indian subcontinent
LBM	lean body mass
LDL	low density lipoprotein
MEND	Mind, Exercise, Nutrition and Do it
MET	metabolic equivalent
MRC	Medical Research Council
MRI	magnetic resonance imaging
NASH	non-alcoholic steatohepatitis
NHANES	National Health and Nutrition Examination Survey (USA)

NICE	National Institute for Health and Clinical Excellence
NIDDM	non-insulin-dependent diabetes mellitus
NIH	National Institutes of Health (USA)
NOF	National Obesity Forum
OSAS	obstructive sleep apnoea syndrome
PA	physical activity
PAL	physical activity level
PCOS	polycystic ovary syndrome
PCT	primary care trust
PE	physical education
PWS	Prader–Willi syndrome
RCGP	Royal College of General Practitioners
RCN	Royal College of Nursing
RCPCH	Royal College of Paediatrics and Child Health
RMR	resting metabolic rate
SES	socioeconomic status
SIGN	Scottish Intercollegiate Guidelines Network
SUFE	slipped upper femoral epiphysis
TLD	Traffic Light Diet
WC	waist circumference
WHO	World Health Organization
WHR	waist : hip ratio

Introduction

Prevalence

Obesity in childhood is not a new problem. It is the extent to which it is occurring which is new and disturbing because of the long-term implications of overweight for later health (Haslam and James 2005). For many years the prevalence of obesity in children in the UK remained fairly static. Since the mid 1980s prevalence has increased virtually every time it is surveyed. For some years the changing situation was difficult to assess and confirm since there were differences in the methods for assessing obesity in childhood in different surveys. Those differences have now been largely resolved (see Chapter 2) but prevalences continue to rise. Table 1.1 shows the changing prevalence of overweight/obesity in English and Scottish children over recent years. Different surveys involve different populations (England and Wales, UK or smaller geographical area; age range) so absolute figures vary, even for studies in the same year, but the trends remain the same. Figure 1.1 indicates how the prevalences of overweight and obesity in girls and boys have changed over the ten years from 1995 to 2004. There are not only more overweight children but those that are overweight seem more overweight with obese children actually outnumbering those only overweight. The prognosis is grim with suggestions of increases of around 300 000 further obese children by 2010 bringing the total to more than 1.7 million (Zaninotto et al. 2006). Currently, there are about 1.25 million overweight and a further 1.4 obese children between 2 and 15 years old in the UK (Zaninotto et al. 2006).

Obesity is not simply a concern about size and appearances. Table 1.2 outlines some of the major health and social implications of obesity, both those affecting overweight children and those that have effects in later life. These effects explain why burgeoning obesity has quite suddenly become an issue for governmental as well as medical concern. Unfortunately it seems to be taking time for that concern to translate into effective preventive and therapeutic action (Haslam and James 2005).

Table 1.1. Percentage prevalence of childhood overweight and obesity in UK 1974–2004[a,b]

Year	1974	1984	1994	1996–7	1998–9	2001/2	2001/2	2003	2004
Boys				5–10 years				2–10 years	
Overweight	11.3	9.8	12.7	16.2	19.7	21.7	22.6	29.7	30.5
Obese	1.8	1.2	2.4	3.4	4.7	5.6	6.0	15.1	15.9
Girls				5–10 years				2–10 years	
Overweight	9.6	10.0	14.4	17.5	19.1	22.6	23.7	25.8	27.7
Obese	1.3	1.8	2.7	4.3	5.3	5.2	6.6	12.4	12.8

[a] Stamatakis et al. (2005).
[b] Health Survey for England 2004 (2006).

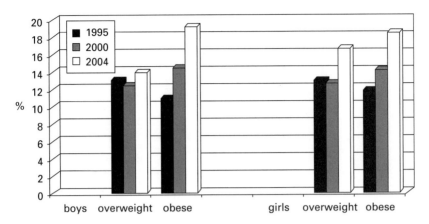

Figure 1.1 Prevalences of overweight and obesity in English boys and girls aged 2–15, 1995–2004. (From Health Survey for England 2004, 2006.)

It is not only in affluent western countries that childhood obesity has become a noticeable concern (Popkin and Doak 1998). Although for the most part at a much lower prevalence, obesity at all ages is becoming increasingly common amongst the more prosperous and urbanized in many of the less developed countries (Araujo *et al.* 2006). It is disappointing that some of these countries have moved from a situation where undernutrition in childhood was a major concern to one where there is now the problem of overnutrition without a noticeable period of normal growth and fatness in between (Popkin and Gordon-Larsen 2004). The disadvantages of westernization have too readily overwhelmed these societies. This creates an interesting pattern of obesity prevalence which has been recognized for many years, namely that obesity tends to be most common amongst the rich in less developed countries and amongst the socioeconomically disadvantaged in more affluent countries. There are exceptions to such a generalization of course, one example being the high prevalence of obesity amongst children of affluent families in some of the rich oil states of the Middle East (Musaiger *et al.* 2000; Mohammadpour-Ahranjani *et al.* 2004). In the UK, differences in prevalence associated with socioeconomic status (SES) are less obvious in children than in adults (see later).

Why is overweight/obesity so prevalent today?

Genes versus environment

Obesity is almost certainly a combination of genetic and environmental causes. Single gene disorders leading to deficient leptin production, insatiable

Table 1.2. Some immediate and later consequences of overweight/obesity in childhood.

Consequences	Type of problem	When and how	Examples
Health consequences	Physical	Immediate	Physical discomfort
			Intertrigo
			Orthopaedic problems
			Breathlessness on exertion
			Asthma
		Adolescent or adult life	Reduced average lifespan
			Type 2 diabetes
			Metabolic syndrome
			Orthopaedic problems:
			Blount's syndrome
			Slipped upper femoral epiphysis
			Increased risk of some cancers
	Emotional	Immediate	Teasing and bullying
			Embarrassment especially with PE
			Low self-esteem
			School underachievement
		Later	Low self-esteem
			Depression
			Professional underachievement
Social consequences	Discrimination	Employment	Less likely to succeed in job
			Less likely to marry successfully
			Less likely to achieve promotion
		Health insurance	More expensive or unobtainable

Physical		Public transport often not sized for obese
		Fashionable clothing may be unavailable in very large sizes
		Public toilet cubicles/public transport seats/theatre seats etc. too small
Economic	For individual	
	General expenses	Greater costs for clothing, transport, insurance etc.
	Employment	Working below ability leading to low wages
	For community	
	Health service costs	Massive costs to public and private health care from problems attributable to or exacerbated by obesity
	Infrastructural costs	Redesigning public buildings and related facilities
		Public transport/theatres etc. cannot accommodate previous numbers because of greater individual space required

appetite and intractable obesity more or less from birth do exist but are very rare (Farooqi and O'Rahilly 2000). (Leptin is a hormone produced by adipose tissue and is involved in the regulation of appetite and energy metabolism.) Across the world certain ethnic groups, most famously the Pima Indians (Schultz *et al.* 2006), seem at particular risk of overweight/obesity in environments of relative affluence. If we look at other ethnic groups in Europe and North America, it can be difficult to assess populations separately from the implications of their social environments. However Saxena *et al.* (2004) concluded that independent of SES, children of Afro-Caribbean ethnic origin and girls of Pakistani origin in Britain had increased risk of obesity. Boys with family origins in India and Pakistan had increased risk of overweight also. Adults from the Indian subcontinent (ISC) are recognized as at greater risk of the co-morbidities of obesity than white British. There is some evidence that this increased risk may be discernable in children as young as 8 years (Whincup *et al.* 2002). Thus the concern excited by overweight amongst children of UK families originating from the ISC should be greater than for white British children.

Obesity occurring in families is very common (Garn 1976; Poskitt and Cole 1978). How much this is due to common genes or common environments is debated but the explanation for today's prevalence of overweight/obesity would seem to be due to changes in the environment acting on individuals with some susceptibility to overweight (Griffiths and Payne 1976; Romon *et al.* 2005). How much genetic predispositions to the co-morbidities of obesity rather than the obesity itself are also influential is again debated (Bjorntorp 2001). It seems unlikely that there has been sufficient recent change in the gene pool to account for the prevalence of obesity across the world today. Since we can do little to alter the genetic background to the present epidemic our interest will concentrate on environmental changes.

Programming

The past 20 years have seen an explosion of research into the relation of events in fetal and early postnatal life to disease processes in later childhood and adult life, the so-called 'programming' of chronic non-communicable diseases. Some of these studies relate to the 'thrifty phenotype hypothesis' which links prenatal and perinatal events to later obesity and non-insulin-dependent (type 2) diabetes mellitus (Hales *et al.* 1992; Barker 1994). However the results from different studies often seem in conflict (Huxley *et al.* 2002; Singhal *et al.* 2003). Thus low birth weight infants with rapid catch-up growth in early infancy can seem particularly prone to develop overweight/obesity later (Ong *et al.* 2000; Yajnik *et al.* 2003). It is the catch-up growth that is important since studies without documented catch-up growth indicate low birth weight is more likely to be associated with relatively short stature, underweight and, in women, low fat mass (Li *et al.* 2003). In other studies high birth weight infants are also at risk of later obesity (Baird *et al.* 2005) although Parsons *et al.* (2001) conclude this association may be determined more by the influence of maternal weight and body mass index (BMI) than specifically by the birth weight. Aspects common to many of the growth related factors suggested as risk factors for obesity are good growth (high birth weight) and evidence of ability for rapid growth (postnatal catch-up growth). Since overweight almost inevitably involves a period of accelerated growth, are these factors just showing what must be an inevitable precursor of obesity or are they acting as drivers or programmers of later obesity (Lucas *et al.* 1999)?

Some of these programming events have particularly strong links with the co-morbidities of obesity/overweight such as coronary heart disease (Eriksson *et al.* 1999), type 2 diabetes and hypertension (Barker 1994). However there is not unanimity of view (Huxley and Neil 2004). Social circumstances, country of residence, gender, postnatal nutrition and health of subjects and a wide range of other factors may confound some studies.

Programming studies have led to greatly increased understanding of the development of non-infectious chronic disease. Whilst the findings are very relevant to some overweight/obese, it is difficult to see these studies explaining the high prevalence of overweight/obesity in childhood and adult life that we see today. Birth weights are higher than in the past. Severe intrauterine growth retardation is probably less common than in the past because it is recognized antenatally and affected infants may be delivered prematurely before growth retardation has had its full effect. There are more low and very low birth weight infants surviving than in the past. Some of these infants do have rapid early growth and may become fat in the first year, particularly if early nutritional supplementation to encourage early weight gain continues once the infant is progressing well. However this latter group forms a very small proportion of the infants born today and cannot begin to account for the epidemic increase in overweight/obesity. Early infant feeding, although rarely following the recommended exclusive breast feeding until the age of 6 months, is markedly more physiological than in the late 1960s when formula milks had quite dangerous composition, introduction to non-milk, non-formula foods was common in the first month of life and overweight and obese infants were very common (Taitz 1971; Shukla *et al.* 1972). Breast feeding, although not nearly as prevalent as would be wished, is significantly more common and of longer mean duration than was the case in UK 40 years ago. All these changes might suggest – from programming findings – that obesity would be on the decline. Yet, despite infant formulas being refined to a composition in many ways similar to breast milk and despite breast feeding statistics improving, the prevalence of overweight and obese children has increased.

This book is concerned with the management of children who are, for whatever reason, now overweight or obese. It focuses on presenting practical approaches to management rather than on extensively exploring the under-lying pathophysiological changes. In this respect, the fascinating work on the fetal and infant origins of disease in later childhood and adult life seem of minor practical clinical relevance here. The risk for type 2 diabetes for example may relate to happenings before birth but the reduction of that risk depends on what happens to that child now and in the future. Whilst catch-up growth may be a critical feature in pre-obese growth for some infants, we believe the main emphasis in infancy should be on the promotion of good weaning practices and healthy lifestyles as children mature. One of us showed many years ago that most infants fat in the first months of life slim down by 5 years old (Poskitt and Cole 1977). The present obesogenic environment may have reduced the chances of fat infants slimming, but it is difficult to blame this on early programming since the infantile obesity seen in the late 1960s was much more prevalent than today. The second 6 months of life – the time of weaning and increasing weight bearing activity for the infant – seems much more critical for the development of persistent obesity (Tate *et al.* 2006). Trying to control weight gain, other than making sure feeding is appropriate, in very young infants brings a risk of affecting the overall nutrition of infants whose unusual patterns of growth may only reflect the expression of genetic potential for growth released from intrauterine constraints.

Family history

The one common risk factor in more or less all studies of the epidemiology of obesity in childhood is a family history of obesity (Poskitt and Cole 1978; Garn and Lavelle 1985). Some 70 to 80 per cent of obese children have one obese parent and 20 to 40 per cent have both parents obese. Whilst children and parents usually share an environment and thus some of this obesity is environmentally induced, studies in the 1960s and 1970s on mono- and dizygotic twins (Børjeson 1976), on twins reared apart (Stunkard *et al.* 1990) and on adopted children (Stunkard *et al.* 1986) suggested that the genetic predisposition to obesity was more dominant than the shared family envir-onment in determining body size. More recent studies show the same find-ings in that adiposity correlations were still greater for monozygotic twins than dizygotic twins even when reared apart (Bodurtha *et al.* 1990). All these studies took place in less obesogenic environments than exist in many societies today. Environmental effects may be more pervasive and influential for relative adiposity in our present obesogenic world.

Changes in the genetic pool cannot explain the rapid increase in obesity in UK in recent years – the change in prevalence has been too rapid – but there seems no doubt that the genetic make-up of some individuals makes them more at risk of obesity in modern society than others. Recent changes would seem to show no longer is it just those with strong predisposition to obesity who are at risk but also those with presumably less strong predisposition to obesity. Some of these latter also progress to obesity thus creating the prevalence we experience today. However, data from France (Romon *et al.* 2005) show that in a population of children with increasing prevalence of overweight, those on the lowest centiles of fatness only show increases in fatness if they are of low SES. In other words those children with higher SES and little predisposition to obesity seem less affected by environmental changes – but why? Do we need to focus more on why some children/adults stay slim within our obesogenic society rather than collect yet more data on the obese in the search for specific precipitating factors to explain their condition?

We do not know if the genetic predisposition (or not) to obesity relates to inherited differences in basal metabolic rates (BMR) which do exist (Bogardus *et al.* 1986), appetite control (Cutting *et al.* 1999), utilization of food energy (Griffiths and Payne 1976; Bouchard *et al.* 1990), aspects of activity or a myriad of other possible causes. Probably all these and other factors are relevant to some cases but separation of the genetic and environmental contributions to obesity from amongst these contributors remains difficult. Parents, at least in early childhood years, are usually the main carers and providers of food, exercise and lifestyle. They share genes and environment with their children.

Socioeconomic status

Socioeconomic circumstances may provide more important determinants of obesity in adult life than in childhood. Indeed, studies from Denmark suggest it may be the environment rather than the family's own SES which promotes obesity in the young adults (Lissau-Lund-Sorenson and Sorensen 1992). In UK studies, adult obesity seems to result from a combination of genetic predisposition, childhood environment and later life experiences (Brummer and McCarthy 2001; Viner and Cole 2005). The effects of SES on prevalence vary according to the place of study, the age of the children studied and perhaps the date of the study. In both North America and Norway overweight/obesity prevalences seem higher in children of poor families although the overall prevalence is much lower in Norway than in North America (Phipps *et al.* 2006). In England the socioeconomic effects on overweight seem less obvious in some (Viner and Cole 2005) but not all studies (Stamatakis *et al.* 2005). Socioeconomic differences on prevalence may be more prominent in Scotland (Armstrong *et al.* 2003). Further, Jebb *et al.* (2003) found children in families from the ISC were four times more likely to be overweight than white British children. In this study the prevalence of obesity was significantly higher in children from social class IV and V than in those from classes I–III and amongst children in Wales and Scotland than those from England. Viner and Cole (2005) found obesity more likely to present in adult life in women with poorer employment and relationships but childhood obesity did not relate to adult socioeconomic circumstances, income, years of schooling, educational attainment, relationships or psychological morbidity.

Energy balance

As we shall discuss in later chapters, obesity in those with otherwise normal growth and no recognized underlying condition must arise when energy intakes exceed energy expenditures. How has energy balance changed to account for the dramatic and rapid increase in obesity in childhood in so many countries over the past 20 years? Specific habits may be responsible for obesity in individuals but the worldwide increased prevalence seems to relate to a range of changes in many modern societies which together create an overall obesogenic environment.

Energy intakes

In the UK, data on energy intakes over the past 50 years suggest children eat less in terms of energy (calories) than they did 50 years ago (Gregory *et al.* 1995; Gregory and Lowe 2000) but they are eating very differently (see later Table 9.3). The variety of foods now available, the availability of foods, advertising pressures and increased affluence for many have changed what is eaten in many cases. Societal attitudes to the way we eat have also changed. As an example, eating in the street is much more acceptable than it was in the past, when many children were told it was something that 'one did not do'. Relative affluence, available food, pressure from advertising and what appear to be reduced energy requirements have enabled families not only to feed their children adequately but too well. We discuss these issues further in Chapter 9.

Energy expenditures

If the evidence for children's energy intakes being greater than in the past is not strong and yet children are fatter, the conclusion must be that energy expenditures have decreased. This certainly seems the case in the UK. Children and their parents are more reliant on cars, walk or cycle less, and in many cases indulge in little formal physical activity. The introduction of the National Curriculum in 1990 resulted in schools focusing less on physical education (PE) and games but this situation does seem to be beginning to reverse. People are also more sedentary. Twenty-four-hour coverage and widespread ownership of television, DVDs and computers create the probability that enjoyable small screen entertainment is available 'around the clock'.

Early feeding

The quality and quantity of infant nutrition are often cited in relation to the development of later overweight and obesity. The current increased prevalence of overweight/obesity in preschool children – previously an age with very low prevalence of obesity – might indicate that changed feeding in young children is partly responsible for some of the obesity epidemic. Breast feeding is often stated as protecting against obesity in children (von Kries et al. 1999; Bergmann et al. 2003). However the data are not consistent (Clifford 2003; Araujo et al. 2006; Burdette et al. 2006) perhaps partly because 'breast feeding' has no specific definition (how exclusive? how long?). Further, it is difficult to have truly comparable groups of breast fed and non breast fed infants since the prevalence of breast feeding is heavily linked with a variety of social and aspirational factors in the lives of mothers. The intimacy of the process of breast feeding may introduce all sorts of specific maternal–child emotional (as well as physical) interactions which could influence later nurture significantly. It would seem likely that mothers who exclusively breast feed their infants for some months acquire a sensitivity to when their infants need food, are satisfied, are looking for comfort rather than food, more readily than might be the case for those formula feeding from a bottle. Such sensitivity could affect mothers' later interpretations of whether their children are hungry and how much food they need, thus making the difference between normal and excessive weight gain. The arguments are perhaps spurious. Breast feeding has many advantages for both mothers and infants and we support exclusive breast feeding in early life irrespective of whether or not it is protective against childhood obesity.

Weaning

Data are more suggestive that a critical period for the development of obesity is the weaning period, that is from around 6 months of age onwards, when 'solid' foods are being introduced and eating habits for mixed diets are being established, rather than the earlier exclusive breast or formula feeding period (Tate et al. 2006). Food behaviours learned at weaning may influence later eating habits and food preferences in ways which could reduce or increase risks for later obesity. The adiposity rebound (AR) is discussed in Chapter 2. We prefer to give emphasis to ensuring that the physiological slimming which precedes the AR and takes place between 6 and 24 months of age, is allowed to take place through the development of appropriate diet and activity in

Table 1.3. Risk factors for childhood obesity

Specific gene defects leading to leptin deficiency	
Ethnicity	Pima Indians; Polynesians
	Children in families from the ISC living in UK
Family history of obesity	Parents, siblings
Other inconsistently associated factors	Low socioeconomic circumstances
	High birth weight
	Low birth weight
	Maternal smoking in pregnancy and rapid catch-up growth
	Not breast fed
	Rapid catch-up growth in infancy
	Early adiposity rebound

young children. The risk of the AR precipitating obesity immediately afterwards should be less if the children have slimmed down and are being encouraged to follow healthy lifestyles.

There are many factors that have been associated with increased or decreased prevalence of obesity in children (Reilly *et al.* 2005). Table 1.3 lists some of these. With the exception of a family history of obesity mentioned above, none seems a consistent predictor of obesity. Further, when looking at risk factors for obesity, we should try to distinguish factors that drive obesity from factors that are inevitable associations (Lucas *et al.* 1999). As mentioned earlier, relative weight at one age cannot be totally independent of previous relative weight for age and height. Rapid weight gain must take place at some time if a child is to become overweight/obese. Thus it is not surprising that these features are associated with the development of obesity later. Slow weight gainers would seem extremely unlikely (assuming children have normal linear growth) ever to become overweight.

A recent paper (Keith *et al.* 2006) discusses a range of putative explanations for the obesity epidemic in addition to excessive energy intake and insufficient activity. These include sleep deficit and needlessly high environmental temperatures in the home (which again we discuss in Chapter 8) as well as other explanations mostly of more relevance to adult than childhood obesity. All these possible contributors to the secular increase in overweight/obesity need further investigation and research if they are to seem convincing explanations. Nevertheless, they provide evidence for the multiplicity of reasons thought relevant to the rise of obesity at all ages and in many societies today.

Table 1.4. Some recent reports and guidelines on obesity: UK and WHO

Organization	Title	Date	Source
National Audit Office	*Tackling Obesity in England*	2001	London: National Audit Office
British Nutrition Foundation	*Obesity: Report of the British Nutrition Task Force*, 2nd edn	2003	London: British Nutrition Foundation
Scottish Intercollegiate Guideline Network (SIGN)	*Management of Obesity in Children and Young People*, Guideline No. 69	2003	www.sign.ac.uk/guidelines
Association for the Study of Obesity, MRC Human Nutrition Research and London School of Hygiene and Tropical Medicine	*A Leaner Fitter Future: Options for Action*	2003	www.mrc-hnr.cam.ac.uk/downloads/aLeanerFitterFuture.pdf
Department of Health	*Choosing Health*	2004	London: The Stationery Office
Royal College of Physicians, Royal College of Paediatrics and Child Health and Faculty of Public Health	*Storing up Problems: The Medical Case for a Slimmer Nation*	2004	London: Royal College of Physicians
House of Commons Health Committee	*Obesity: Third Report of Session 2003/4*	2004	London: The Stationery Office
National Institute for Health and Clinical Excellence (NICE)	*Obesity: Guidance on the Prevention, Identification, Assessment and Management of Overweight and Obesity in Adults and Children*	2006	www.nice.org.uk/guidance/CG43
International Obesity Task Force, Report to WHO	*Obesity in Children and Young People: A Crisis in Public Health*	2004	Obesity Reviews 2004 (Lobstein *et al.* 2004)

What is being done?

The last ten years have seen a plethora of reports on obesity and national guidelines on its management in UK and abroad. Table 1.4 lists some of these. Despite all the public and governmental concern about the epidemic of childhood obesity and despite a massive increase in the amount of research taking place, facilities for managing obese children in the UK remain few and far between. Obesity management has little drama to appeal to enthusiastic health care practitioners (HCPs) keen to make dramatic changes to people's health and lives. Management of obesity is widely considered ineffective making it an unattractive work choice. Few want to embark on projects that seem doomed to failure. The prevailing public attitude is that obesity is not a medical issue but something brought on by the individual or, for a child, by the individual's parents. It is up to those affected to put this right themselves. If they cannot manage it, this indicates personal failings. Such attitudes do not acknowledge the enormous pressures the modern environment places on families. It is too easy in the modern world to act in ways which lead those with susceptible genetic make-ups to overweight and obesity. Such attitudes also overlook the costs to individual families, the economy and health services of dealing with the social and economic consequences of obesity. This is something governments are beginning to recognize. As Table 1.2 shows, the obese are not only more likely to die young, be infertile, at risk of complications when pregnant, or to be unable to work in later life because of disabilities related to their obesity, but they are less likely to succeed at school, at work or in marriage (Haslam *et al.* 2006). The more our population becomes obese, the more there is a risk that a significant proportion of our nation will underachieve. It is only pragmatic that we do what we can to reduce this waste of economic productivity and of aspiration (McCarthy 2004; Haby *et al.* 2006).

Ideally effective preventive programmes (see Chapter 13) are the way forward to managing the obesity epidemic since prevention should be easier to implement than weight control and reduction of fat once children are burdened with obesity. However, as we stated earlier, there are currently well over a million children in the UK who are already obese (Zaninotto *et al.* 2006). If they are to avoid living shorter lives than their parents because they are overwhelmed by the complications of obesity this generation of children need help (Olshansky *et al.* 2005; Preston 2005).

In the next few chapters we try to provide a background to childhood obesity. Later chapters make suggestions for what can be done and how this should be done. Imagination, skill and interest are needed by all those concerned so their varied skills, their facilities and their time are used to effect weight change in the child population.

2

How fat is fat? Measuring and defining overweight and obesity

Obesity is an excess of body fat. In adults, values for the 'normal' and 'healthy' amounts of body fat have not been defined although it is recognized that on average men and women differ in the percentage of body weight as fat (%BF) with women being fatter than men. Percentage BF is also under genetic influence and there are ethnic and familial differences in normal fatness. In childhood the proportion of fat to lean tissue in the body not only varies between boys and girls, but also changes with age and physical maturity making it even more difficult to determine what is physiologically normal either for an individual or for a population (Table 2.1).

Even within populations with similar lifestyles, the range of fatness between individuals is wide. Familial tendencies to obesity are probably a mixture of the effects of shared environment and shared genetic inheritance.

Fattening periods

Table 2.1 shows how estimated fatness as %BF varies with age in boys and girls. The absolute values vary with the method used to determine them and in most cases the values were recorded some years ago when the subject population was considerably thinner than now.

Physiologically the age related changes in body composition suggest the body prepares for periods of vigorous growth (early years, puberty and pregnancy) by laying down fat which can then fuel subsequent growth.

Early infancy

Figure 2.1 illustrates the changing fattening and 'stretching' periods of childhood in boys and girls. Between birth and the time when most normal infants double their birth weights (around 4–5 months), the amount of fat in infants' bodies trebles. By around 6 months of age – when the introduction to

Table 2.1. Estimates of percentage body fat (%BF) at different ages in childhood

Age	Widdowson 1971[a] Both sexes	Fomon 1974[b] Boys	Fomon 1974[b] Girls	Rauh and Schumsky 1968[c] Boys	Rauh and Schumsky 1968[c] Girls	McCarthy et al. 2006[d] Boys	McCarthy et al. 2006[d] Girls
26 weeks gestation	1						
Term infant	16	14	15				
4 months		25	25				
12 months		23	24				
5 years				13	15	16	18
10 years				18	20	18	23
15 years				11	23	16	24
18 years				12	25	15	25

[a] Analysis of chemical composition of body.
[b] Derived from total body water estimates.
[c] Derived from skinfold measurements and formula developed from relating skinfolds to total body water.
[d] Derived from bioelectrical impedance measurements.

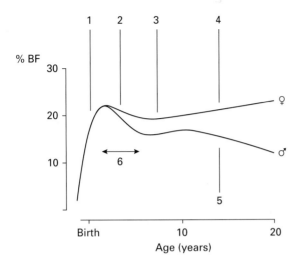

Figure 2.1 Sex and age related changes in percentage body fat (%BF). 1, prenatal and postnatal fattening; 2, weaning period 'stretching'; 3, adiposity rebound; 4, girls: pubertal fattening; 5, boys: pubertal slimming; 6, period of potential early adiposity rebound.

semi-solid and solid foods is recommended – overall rate of weight gain in g/kg per day has slowed dramatically compared with that in the first months. The rate of fat deposition relative to lean tissue deposition has also fallen. Percentage body fat declines gradually until around 5 years of age (Fomon 1974).

Age 5–10 years: the adiposity rebound

From around 5 years old, children begin to increase rates of fat deposition again: the adiposity rebound (AR). If this rebound in fat deposition occurs early (before 5 years of age) children seem at particular risk of persistent obesity (Rolland-Cachera *et al.* 1984). An early AR is thus considered a predetermining factor for persistent obesity although Dietz (1994) has pointed out that children on the higher BMI centiles have earlier AR, so early rebound may only reflect the advanced growth of already heavier children. There may be other explanations for associations between early AR and persistent obesity. Children who fatten when others are showing normal physiological slimming may be children with either strong genetic predisposition to obesity or factors in their lifestyle which vigorously promote fat deposition. If either, or both, of these is present it is not surprising that, at later ages when normal children tend to fatten, those who were already fattening at above normal rates may continue to do so and become overweight or obese. The focus on early AR may have been misplaced. The emphasis should perhaps be on the *earlier adiposity reduction* or stretching. Ensuring that infants move into a slimming phase in the second 6 months of life as their diets change and their weight bearing activities increase could have more impact managing overweight than making gloomy prognostications once an early AR is under way.

Males: pre-puberty

Boys who are growing well but have relatively delayed puberty may continue relatively high rates of fat deposition until their pubertal growth spurt. Some of these boys will become overweight or obese but, if wisely managed, this overweight/obesity should disappear with the growth spurt and the changes in fat deposition and body composition that accompany this (Bogin 1999). In past experience the physiological tendency to lose pre-pubertal fatness as puberty advanced was a useful adjunct to other lifestyle changes in the control of male adolescent overweight/obesity. The present, highly obesogenic, environment may antagonize this natural fall in fatness with late puberty making it unwise to rely on physiological changes alone to control the obesity of adolescent boys.

Boys showing constitutional growth delay with both short stature for age and proportionately low body weight pre-pubertally seem less at risk of overweight than those whose linear growth remains within the normal range despite late maturation.

Females: late puberty

The adolescent growth spurt in girls is smaller, peaks earlier and finishes sooner than in boys (Patton and Viner 2007). Puberty in girls is associated with vigorous fat deposition and girls with early puberty tend to become obese more readily than late maturing girls (Freedman *et al.* 2003). It is not clear how much this is a consequence of overnutrition promoting advanced growth and maturation or of early maturity and cessation of the growth spurt leading to reduced energy needs at a time when the peer group is possibly eating more to support pubertal growth (Pierce and Leon 2005; Kaplowitz 2006). Early maturing girls, even if not overweight at puberty, may benefit from lifestyle advice to avoid later obesity, particularly if they come from families prone to obesity.

Methods of measuring fatness and defining obesity

Table 2.2 lists direct and indirect methods of assessing overweight and obesity. Direct methods of looking at the amount and distribution of fat in

Table 2.2. Methods of assessing %BF and overweight/obesity

Estimation of body fat from magnetic resonance imaging (MRI)
Estimation of body fat from dual X-ray absorptiometry (DEXA)
Estimation of body fat from computerized axial tomography (CT) scanning
Body density: total immersion
Total body water
Total body potassium
Derivation of body fat from bioelectrical impedance
Anthropometry: Skinfold thicknesses
                  Waist circumference
                  Waist : hip circumference ratio
                  Weight and height ratios: BMI

the body by magnetic resonance imaging (MRI), dual X-ray absorptiometry (DEXA) or by computerized tomography (CT) provide very specific information but the costs of equipment, the need for experienced technicians, the lack of availability of equipment outside hospitals and the need for children to lie still for quite long periods together with the X-ray dose in the case of CT, make these methods unsuitable for regular clinical assessment of the obese (Wells and Fewtrell 2006). The X-ray doses used in DEXA are extremely small but the equipment does not show the distribution of fat in the detail of MRI and CT scanning and it has the same disadvantages as MRI and CT scanning in terms of primary care use.

Other methods for assessing fatness either attempt to measure the lean and fat tissue compartments in the body or use measurements such as weight and height or waist circumferences as proxy indicators of fat mass. Table 2.3 outlines issues relating to methods attempting to measure %BF. More details can be obtained from Lobstein *et al.* (2004) and Wells and Fewtrell (2006).

Measuring the proportion of fat in the body

The body can be considered as consisting of various compartments. The simplest model for assessment of obesity is to consider a two-compartment model of fat and lean tissue. Fat tissue is assumed almost free of water, free of potassium and of a lower density than lean tissue. Using these assumptions body composition estimates have been made from measurements of total body water, total body potassium or body density. However, fat and lean tissues are not totally separate in the body. Some essential fat occurs in lean tissues and connective tissue percolates through adipose tissue. Nevertheless these compartment models can give some idea of relative amounts of body fat and are often used to calibrate indirect methods of assessing %BF measurements.

Table 2.3. Methods of assessing body composition

Method	Brief description	Positive points	Negative points	Reference
Magnetic resonance imaging (MRI)	Develops images of adipose and other tissues from which total body fat, %BF and body fat distribution can be assessed.	Very detailed images; can distinguish intra-abdominal from subcutaneous fat.	Expensive equipment. Needs well-trained technicians. Hospital-based equipment. Requires subject to lie still in scanner for about 30 minutes.	Brambilla et al. (2006), Wells and Fewtrell (2006)
Dual X-ray absorptiometry (DEXA)	Equations developed from attenuation of energy from two X-ray doses can be used to estimate total fat and %BF but does not show distribution of fat.	Very low dosage of X-rays used compared with CT scanning.	Expensive equipment. Needs well-trained technicians. Hospital-based equipment. Subject needs to keep still for approximately 20 minutes.	Silva et al. (2006)
Computerized axial tomography (CAT)	High resolution images show distribution of adipose tissue in great detail enabling total body fat, %BF and distribution to be evaluated.	Accurate quantification of intra-abdominal and subcutaneous fat.	Expensive equipment. Needs well-trained technicians. Hospital and research unit based equipment. Requires subject to lie still in scanner for about 30 minutes.	Goran (1998)
Body density	Weighing during total body immersion whilst holding breath. Needs estimate of air in lungs as well.	'Gold standard'.	Bathing costume. Frightening for those not water confident. Cumbersome equipment unsuitable for general practice.	Goran (1998)

Method	Procedure	Advantages	Disadvantages	References
Air displacement plethysmography	Subject sits in enclosed cabinet for less than 5 minutes. Weight recorded at the same time. Displacement of air in chamber in cabinet assesses volume.	Quick, reasonably accurate. Can be adapted for children. If explained well is acceptable to children.	Moderately expensive equipment for primary care. Subject wears tightly fitting costume and tightly fitting cap.	Fields et al. (2002), Wells et al. (2003)
Total body water	Subject given dose of heavy water. After equilibration time, distribution measured and total body water estimated.	Simple, non-invasive. Heavy water can be given orally and distribution estimated from saliva samples.	Expensive. Total body water decreases with age in the first 3 years of life. Unsuitable for primary care.	Wells et al. (2003)
Total body potassium		Non-invasive.	Equipment for measuring ^{40}K expensive and cumbersome. Equipment largely confined to research establishments. Requires being shut for >30 minutes in small chamber. Not suitable for primary care. Calibration needed for size of subject.	Garrow (2005)
Bioelectrical impedance (BI)	Assumes adipose tissue is free of water. Small pain-free current passed through body from electrodes usually attached to limbs	Repeatable results Non-invasive	Results dependent on instrument used, hydration and diet of subject. Circumstances need to be the same at each recording. Value in children under 5 uncertain.	McCarthy et al. (2006), Wells and Fewtrell (2006)

The 'gold standard' method of estimating the body fat component has been underwater weighing to obtain body density and calculating %BF from that. As with most of the methods described in Table 2.3, underwater weighing is impractical for the clinical assessment of fatness in childhood. None of these methods gives any indication of what should be acceptable as 'normal' %BF. Indeed, different methods of assessing %BF and/or percentage lean tissue are likely to measure slightly different body compartments. Each method's results are thus not directly comparable although they should correlate in terms of high or low values.

Recently methods for measuring body density by air displacement plethysmography have been developed. These involve a much quicker and simpler procedures than underwater weighing and seem to have acceptable accuracy. Bioelectrical impedance (BI), another quick and fairly adaptable technique (although its accuracy is sometimes questioned), has also attracted a lot of use because it is non-invasive and some relatively cheap equipment is now on the market.

Possible primary care equipment for measuring body fatness

Measurement of body density: Bod Pod (Life Measurements Inc., Concord, CA)

The Bod Pod (Life Measurements Inc., Concord, CA) is a commercial item which determines body density quickly from weight and body volume and without the paraphernalia of total body immersion. Currently the Bod Pod is probably too bulky and expensive to be part of general primary health care clinic equipment. However, it is simple to use, has a relatively low margin of error (2% is quoted by the manufacturers) and, when the procedures are explained carefully, the paediatric version is usually tolerated by children. These features make the Bod Pod useful for research studies which involve measuring %BF in children and it may come to have wider use.

Measurement of bioelectrical impedance: Tanita (Tanita Corp., Tokyo, Japan)

Bioelectrical impedance estimates of body composition are based on the concept that the electrical conductivities of lean and fat tissue are different. Determining the conduction of a small electrical impulse from one part of the body to another provides a value for tissue resistance. This, together with weight and height, can be used to estimate body composition using equations which are developed on a particular piece of equipment and with an age and sex related population similar to that under study. An adaptation 'advanced dual frequency technology' uses two different electrical frequencies and is thought to give a more accurate representation of body composition. Bioelectrical impedance is quick and simple to use and non-invasive. Modern

Table 2.4. Mean, 85th and 95th centile values of %BF by age measured by bioelectrical impedance

	Boys			Girls		
	Centile			Centile		
Age	50	85	95	50	85	95
5	15.6	18.6	21.4	18.0	21.5	24.3
6	16.0	19.5	22.7	19.1	23.0	26.2
7	16.5	20.4	24.1	20.2	24.5	28.0
8	17.0	21.3	25.5	21.2	26.0	29.7
9	22.2	26.8	22.1	27.2	31.2	32.2
10	17.8	22.8	27.9	22.8	28.2	32.2
11	17.7	23.0	28.3	23.3	28.8	32.8
12	17.4	22.7	27.9	23.5	29.1	33.1
13	16.8	22.0	27.0	23.8	29.4	33.3
14	16.2	21.3	25.9	24.0	29.6	33.6
15	15.8	20.7	25.0	24.1	29.9	33.8
16	15.5	20.3	24.3	24.3	30.1	34.1
17	15.4	20.1	23.9	24.4	30.4	34.4
18	15.4	20.1	23.6	24.6	30.8	34.8

Source: Adapted from McCarthy *et al.* (2006) with permission.

equipment can be obtained which is not enormously expensive and is more or less portable. One such example is produced by Tanita Corp., Tokyo, Japan. The subject stands on special scales and holds on to hand grips to establish electrical connections. The precision for estimates of body fat in children, particularly the very young, is uncertain because, as previously commented, each piece of equipment should be individually calibrated. Calibration needs to be done not only for each piece of equipment but for children's size and age thus making results not readily comparable even within BI studies. With BI, age is an important variable since the water content of a tissue affects impedance. The extracellular fluid content of the body is high at birth compared with that of adults and decreases gradually over childhood although the main decrease (after dramatic changes in the first weeks of life) takes place in the first 3 years (Widdowson 1971). Results are also affected by the body's state of overall hydration and according to manufacturers, by temperature, amount of exercise, menstruation, medical conditions and medications, alcohol, caffeine and bathing habits.

Table 2.4 gives 85th ('overweight') and 95th ('obese') centiles for %BF measured by BI for children 5–18 years of age (McCarthy *et al.* 2006). It is uncertain how applicable these results will be to other estimates of %BF for the reasons discussed above. There are no 'reference' standards for %BF in children.

Body fat distribution and measuring fatness in specific areas

The distribution of body fat in adults and, although less well documented, in children is significant for the risk of later complications of obesity. The typically female 'pear' or gynoid distribution of fat around the hips, thighs and more peripherally presents less risk than more central deposition of fat. The central 'apple' or android distribution, especially when the fat is intra-abdominal, is associated with a variety of risks for the serious complications of obesity (see Chapter 6). This has led to waist circumference receiving attention as a proxy for fat distribution. However, measuring fatness by recording the thickness of superficial fat – skinfolds – has a long history.

Skinfolds

Skinfold calipers (Holtain Ltd., Cresswell, Wales, UK) have been developed for recording the thickness of a skinfold. Skinfolds can be measured anywhere it is possible to raise a fold of skin and underlying subcutaneous tissue although the commonest positions (for which there are site definitions) are over the triceps and biceps muscles, in the subscapular and supra-iliac regions and also over the abdomen and thighs. Children find the 'pincher' appearance of the calipers and the process of measurement frightening and uncomfortable. More importantly perhaps, the calipers are not particularly useful in measuring fat in the obese. It can be difficult to raise a fold in significantly obese individuals, the calipers may gradually slip off the fold and, in some cases, the skinfold is thicker than the gape of the calipers. Thus, although there are some, out of date, age and sex related centiles for triceps and subscapular skinfolds in British children (Tanner and Whitehouse 1975), these do not indicate values for an accepted 'normal' range. We do not find skinfold measurements particularly practical or useful in the assessment of childhood overweight/obesity.

Waist circumference

Measuring waist circumference is a simple, relatively acceptable procedure for both children and adults (McCarthy et al. 2001). There are published centiles for age and sex related values for waist circumferences in children (Harlow Printing Company 2007). In adults a measurement >80 cm in women and >85 cm in men is regarded as providing increased risk for the complications of obesity (Lean et al. 1998). Currently there are no criteria for normal or abnormal values in children. It would seem likely that they would be highly age dependent and probably sex dependent as well.

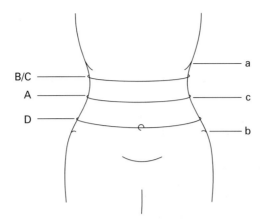

Figure 2.2 Various definitions of waist circumference measurement. Landmarks: a, lower border of costal margin in midaxillary line; b, upper border of iliac crest in midaxillary line; c, horizontal plane midway between a and b. For definitions of waist measurements A, B, C and D see text.

The problem with waist circumference for defining obesity and overweight is lack of consensus over what defines the waist in these circumstances. The following, illustrated in Figure 2.2, are only some of the definitions.

(A) The horizontal circumference at a level halfway between the lower border of the ribs in the mid axillary line and the upper border of the iliac crest in the same vertical line measured at the end of expiration if possible (World Health Organization Expert Committee on Physical Status 1995).

(B) The circumference of the body at the area of noticeable narrowing at the waist (Fitness Canada 1981; Katzmarzyk 2004).

(C) The shortest circumference between ribs and hips when breathing out (National Obesity Forum 2007).

(D) The body circumference at the level of the umbilicus as suggested by the National Obesity Forum for measuring one's own waist. (For some obese with pendulous abdomens the umbilicus may be positioned well below the level normally attributed to the waist.)

These different waist definitions give different results. However, the distribution of the results is very comparable between methods: high results are high and low results low, whichever definition of waist is used (Wang *et al.* 2003; Wang 2006). We recommend the World Health Organization (1995) definition (A) which has the intentions of being an international definition.

Since in adults central, particularly intra-abdominal, obesity is a risk factor for the complications of obesity, waist circumference can be a useful indicator of the distribution of body fat. Sometimes waist : hip ratio (WHR) is used in adults also to indicate relative distribution of fat centrally and peripherally. This ratio has little place in childhood since we know little about how it varies with age. In girls reaching puberty the changes in hip measurements due to pelvic growth can reduce WHR measurements even though waist circumferences remain the same (E. Poskitt, unpublished observation).

Weight and height relationships: BMI

Worldwide, weight for height, which relates weight to a range of expected weights for the child's height, is widely and successfully used to define malnutrition (World Health Organization 1999). However obese prepubertal children are commonly relatively tall for age. Because children tall for age, whether obese or not, tend to have heavier 'build' than those short for age, weight for height is an imprecise way of distinguishing overweight and obese children from their normal fatness, but possibly tall for age, peers.

In adults the body mass index (BMI) is used to define overweight and obesity:

$$\text{BMI} = \text{weight in kg}/(\text{height in m})^2.$$

Table 2.5. BMI classification of nutritional status *in adults*

BMI (kg/m^2)	Status
<18.5	Undernutrition (<16.0 severe malnutrition)
18.5–24.9	Normal weight
>25.0–29.9	Overweight/pre-obese
30.0–34.9	Obese category I
35.0–39.9	Obese category II
40 and over	Obese category III

Source: World Health Organization Expert Committee on Physical Status (1995).

Table 2.5 shows how BMI can be used to define underweight, overweight and obesity in adults.

Body mass index has many advantages as a method of assessing fatness in adults. It is
- simple
- easy to use for categorization of over/underweight
- the same for both sexes in respect of at-risk values for adults
- non-invasive
- acceptable to subjects

- inexpensive
- consistent and repeatable for results
- relatively free of inter-observer variability
- correlated on a population basis with risk of morbidity and mortality although recent large studies have questioned the validity of this long held interpretation (Yusuf *et al.* 2005)

But

- BMI does not measure fat
- values indicating 'at risk of complications' in non-white adults are different from those for white adults
- BMI values vary non-linearly with age in children.

The three last points are important. In modern westernized society most adults with high BMI are excessively fat. However there are individuals whose musculature is very well developed in whom a high BMI can be associated with normal or even low fatness. Such individuals, adults or children, are usually fairly obvious to the observer either by their lifestyles or their obviously muscular appearance. Recognition that adults from the ISC and possibly elsewhere are at risk of the complications of obesity at lower BMI values than Europeans (Jafar *et al.* 2006) raises the question whether BMI should be reviewed for other ethnic groups and, of course, questions whether there should also be different values for UK children from different ethnic groups (Whincup *et al.* 2002).

Recording BMI is cheap and simple. Robust and reliable weighing scales that weigh up to at least 125 kg, scales weighing up to 20 kg suitable for weighing children under 2 years old who may not be prepared to stand on scales; a stadiometer (measures height) suitable for children, a length-measuring board for children under 2 years old (measured lying down), a pocket calculator, and personnel who understand how to measure children accurately (see Chapter 5), are all that are needed.

The variation of BMI with age is the main difficulty in using this measurement in childhood. Body mass index centiles for age have been published and are now widely available (Harlow Printing Company 2007) and their use is being encouraged. Nevertheless there is no good clinical evidence for where cut-off points between normal and abnormal BMI should lie at any age in childhood. This problem has not been fully resolved but Table 2.6 lists some of the criteria used to define overweight and obesity from centile cut-off points in childhood.

The International Obesity Task Force (IOTF) definition for overweight/ obesity in children (Cole *et al.* 2000) creates continuity between the definitions of obesity in childhood and in adult life by choosing overweight and obesity cut-offs as the centiles which trace back in age from the centiles which mark the adult cut-off points for overweight and obesity of 25 kg/m^{2}and 30 kg/m^2 at the age of 18 years. Table 2.7 gives these cut-off points for age in

Table 2.6. Centile (Z score)[a] classifications of BMI cut-off for definition of overweight/obesity in children

| | Centile (Z score)[a] | | Growth standards used | Users | Reference |
	Overweight	Obesity[b]			
1990 UK BMI reference charts[c]	>85th (>1.04)	>95th (>1.64)	UK	Health Survey for England 2002 UK epidemiological and research practice	Scottish Intercollegiate Guidelines Network (2003)
1990 UK BMI reference charts[c]	91st (>1.33)	98th (>2.00)	UK	UK clinical practice UK BMI centile charts	Royal College of Paediatrics and Child Health (2002); Scottish Intercollegiate Guidelines Network (2003)
Six countries reference charts[d]	~ 91st (>1.33)	~98th (>2.00)	Children in UK, Hong Kong, Singapore, Brazil, France,	International comparison; research; clinical publications	Cole et al. (2000)
NIH[e]	>85th (>1.04)	>95th (>1.64)	NHANES I	Practice in USA	Must et al. (1991)
CDC[f]	>85th (>1.04)	>95th (>1.64)	CDC	USA	Must and Anderson (2006)

[a] Z score or SD score $= (V - M)/S$ where V = individual value, M = mean value for age and sex and S = standard deviation (SD) for that mean value. Positive and negative numbers indicate above and below average values respectively for the measurement.
[b] In USA ≥85th centile is classified as 'at risk of overweight' and ≥95th centile as overweight.
[c] Cole et al. (1995).
[d] Cole et al. 2000.
[e] www.cdc.gov/nchs/nhanes.htm.
[f] www.cdc.gov/growthcharts.

Table 2.7. Cut-off age and sex related BMI values on centile equivalent of 25 kg/m² and 30 kg/m² at age 18 years

Age	Boys ≡ BMI 25	Boys ≡ BMI 30	Girls ≡ BMI 25	Girls ≡ BMI 30
2	18.4	20.1	18.0	19.8
3	17.9	19.6	17.6	19.4
4	17.6	19.3	17.3	19.3
5	17.4	19.3	17.1	19.3
6	17.6	19.8	17.3	19.8
7	17.9	20.6	17.8	20.6
8	18.4	21.6	18.3	21.6
9	19.1	22.8	19.1	22.8
10	19.8	24.0	19.9	24.0
11	20.6	25.1	20.7	25.1
12	21.2	26.0	21.7	26.7
13	21.9	26.8	22.6	27.8
14	22.6	27.6	23.3	28.6
15	23.3	28.3	23.9	29.1
16	23.9	28.9	24.4	28.9
17	24.6	29.4	24.7	29.4
18	25	30	25	30

Source: Adapted from Cole *et al.* (2000) with permission

children between 2 and 18 years (Cole *et al.* 2000). There have been suggestions (Chinn and Rona 2001) that a later age for the links with adult BMI, $19\frac{1}{2}$ for example, would give better sensitivities to the definitions of obesity and overweight. Several reports of studies using the IOTF definition suggest it is very specific in that it is largely successful in selecting only children who appear on other grounds to be obese. However it is not very sensitive in that a significant proportion of children do not achieve this cut-off point even though, on clinical examination, they appear overfat. Nevertheless the IOTF definition has been adopted by several scientific journals for presentation of data on overweight and obesity.

Body mass index centile charts for UK children are available (Harlow Printing Company 2007). The appropriate cut-off point for definition of overweight and obesity in individuals in the clinical situation has been debated. However both the National Institute for Health and Clinical Excellence (NICE) (2007) and the Scottish Intercollegiate Guidelines Network (SIGN) (2003) recommend the 91st centile as cut-off for overweight and the 98th centile as cut-off for obesity on UK reference charts. Others use the 85th and 95th centiles for age for overweight and obesity (Table 2.6) and these cut-off points are recommended by NICE (2007) and SIGN (2003) for epidemiological purposes since it is important that epidemiological data are comparable across studies. These are the centiles set as target cut-off points used in the relevant Public Service Agreement to halt the year-on-year increase in obesity prevalence in 2–10-year-olds in the UK.

By using centile positions for their definition, all these criteria presume the same proportion of overweight and obese at all ages in a population of children – something which is almost certainly not the case. Studies of obesity prevalence in childhood show distributions similar to the patterns of relative fatness with age suggesting the tendency of some children to fatten excessively when there is already physiological fattening. Nevertheless the great advantage of BMI centiles for assessing overweight and obesity is that, apart from being non-invasive, cheap and reliable, they provide a common definition which allows data from different studies to be compared – something often impossible in the past when each study tended to define obesity in its own way. Use of the various definitions of overweight and obesity from the BMI centiles is still in early stages. With more experience we may begin to appreciate the advantages and the limitations of the methodology and of the various BMI criteria for defining childhood overweight and obesity.

The BMI value itself is unaffected by the reference standards used in its evaluation since BMI is based on the actual weight and height of a child. However the BMI values forming the centiles in charts or tables will be determined by the population from which the heights and weights were derived. Currently British standards for BMI (Cole *et al.* 1995) are based on 1995 UK growth centiles – a group of children measured in 1990 (Freeman *et al.* 1995). Body mass index centiles should not be updated since, in a population with increasing obesity, this could be confusing and would obscure the true level of obesity in the population. Whether overweight and obesity should be assessed more from international standards by using growth charts such as those produced by the World Health Organization (WHO) is being questioned. Ultimately it is the BMI values in kg/m^2 used as cut-off points which matter. The points suggested by IOTF are determined more by adult criteria for dangerous BMI than any concept of childhood growth. Other cut-off points may have logic but no *clinical* justification at the time of writing (Reilly 2006).

No cut-off should be absolute. A child who has a high BMI for age (e.g. >95th centile) is likely to benefit from some help with weight control (Reilly 2006). A child who looks obese may well be significantly fat even if not meeting the obesity cut-off point since, as we have indicated, the sensitivity of the method seems rather low.

Since determining definitions of overweight and obesity from BMI charts is somewhat confused, considerable clinical judgement is necessary when assessing children's nutritional status. For borderline children whose BMIs fall between the various cut-off points of overweight for example, a single measurement on a child may leave the diagnosis uncertain if the child does not appear clinically very fat. However, a second measurement a month or so later may clarify the position. If the child's BMI 'growth curve' is crossing centiles upwards and is already over the 75th centile, undesirable fattening is likely to be taking place and child and family deserve advice in this respect. If only weight and height are being charted and not BMI, concern should arise if the weight is accelerating upwards across centiles in a way not paralleled by changes in the height centile position.

From September 2006, British children in Reception and Year 6 classes will have their heights and weights measured and BMI calculated. The problem is then what to do with the findings (Westwood *et al.* 2007). However it may be that as a result of these population recordings we shall be able to develop BMI criteria for overweight/obesity in the British population at different ages.

Recommendations

- We recommend that, in clinical practice, a child's nutritional status is estimated from weight and height and calculating BMI which is then plotted on a centile chart (Harlow Printing Company 2007) both for future reference and for evaluating current state of normal or overweight. Alternatively the BMI can be checked against tables of absolute values for the BMI cut-off points at a particular age such as shown in Table 2.7 (IOTF cut-offs for overweight and obesity). We recommend however using the UK BMI centiles with cut-off points for overweight and obesity at the 91st centile and above for overweight and the 98th centile and above for obesity.

- If some estimate of %BF is available we recommend caution when interpreting a single measurement against centiles of McCarthy *et al.* (2006) unless the equipment and methodology used is the same as that used to collect their data. Whatever the reliability of estimates of %BF, values which are changing over time in excess of that suggested by the figures given in Table 2.4 should highlight the likelihood of present, or developing, overweight and obesity. Likewise upward changes in the centile or *Z* scores (for explanation of *Z* scores see footnote to Table 2.6) of BMIs or other estimates of fatness are the most significant indicators of how obesity may be developing or increasing. For adolescents the stage of pubertal development should be included in any evaluation of what is happening to fatness or BMI since early developers may show the fattening that goes with female puberty (for example) at an age when fattening would not otherwise be expected.

- We recommend that every assessment for overweight/obesity is accompanied by clinical observation. Does the child look too fat? (It is important to remember that the overall high prevalence of overweight in childhood today has resulted in many people now equating overfat children with normal weight.) At present the methods for defining overweight/obesity in childhood are likely to exclude a significant proportion of children who would benefit from efforts to control their weight. Provided the advice given to such children is balanced lifestyle change rather than drastic dieting, children who are borderline overweight are unlikely to be harmed by recommendations for changes to healthier lifestyles.

- Weight changes alone can hint at developing obesity. However weight increases naturally with linear growth. Thus an increase in weight can be associated with a falling BMI and reducing fatness if this increase is at a slower rate than would be expected physiologically. Weight changes can only be used to assess overweight and obesity if matched against what is happening to height. A rapidly increasing weight crossing the weight centiles upwards but not paralleled by a similar height increase upwards across the centiles suggests developing overweight/obesity.

- We do not recommend using weight and height alone instead of BMI for assessment of overweight/obesity although plotting these on centile values for age charts can be informative and helpful to show parents.

3

Where should overweight/obese children be managed?

Management of overweight and obesity in childhood or in adult life begins within the home. For those who find it easy – for whatever reason – to control their weight gain, changes in energy intake and output initiated from home may be all that are necessary to regain normal weight and fatness (Poskitt 2002). For those who need more support than can be provided within the family environment the questions then arise where and by whom should help be provided?

In the UK, policies for the management of the obese child have not been widely developed although there are some guidelines for primary and secondary care (Royal College of Paediatrics and Child Health (RCPCH) 2002; Scottish Intercollegiate Guidelines Network (SIGN) 2003; National Institute for Health and Clinical Excellence (NICE) 2006). There are few paediatricians with specialist experience in managing obese children. In the community and in hospitals the problem is much the same – who has the experience, skills, time, interest and suitable facilities to provide effective support and care for overweight children and their families?

Who should manage these children?

Most obese children are not 'ill' in the usual sense. Should they be managed within the health services at all? More and more obese children are now being recognized with co-morbidities of obesity. The potential medical consequences of uncontrolled obesity with the prevalence found in the west today are monumental. It is incumbent upon those involved with the health of children to ensure there are facilities for these children and that the facilities are both appropriate and effective. Yet there is no strong evidence to suggest that any particular facility for obese children is superior to others. What is on offer is so widely variable that comparisons are barely possible.

Who should run what sort of facility?

The most important attributes for those developing facilities for managing obesity/overweight children would seem to be:
- enthusiasm for tackling the problem of child obesity
- time to talk with and advise children and families
- paediatric experience or child-centred professional experience
- basic clinical knowledge about obesity
- basic knowledge about nutrition and physical activity
- understanding of child growth and development
- sensitivity to child–parent interactions and family contextual factors
- access to a centre of referral for children with significant medical, psychosocial or developmental problems
- access to a place to hold the 'clinic'.

Of these attributes the most important are time, enthusiasm and empathy. Professionals with only little nutritional knowledge could be supported by paediatric dietetic services. The individual running the 'clinic' need not be medical but needs access to paediatric advice and support when required. A full clinical history and examination (Chapter 5) can be carried out initially by a paediatrician or a general practitioner with sound paediatric experience before the child is referred for obesity management.

Where?

Table 3.1 outlines advantages and disadvantages of some of the venues currently used for management of childhood obesity. The problem of overweight/obesity may first be raised with the family, or by the family, in the general practitioner's surgery or to the practice nurse. Sometimes it is the school nurse who introduces the family to the idea that the child's weight is a problem. Whether management continues in the surgery, in some community weight control programme or in a hospital paediatric unit is largely determined by what is available locally.

Multidisciplinary clinics are sometimes suggested as the answer to the management of obese children (Flodmark *et al.* 1993). Children are reviewed and advised by paediatrician, psychologist, dietician, physical activity specialist, education psychologist and others, usually within a hospital paediatric unit. Results are not significantly better from such clinics but the multidisciplinary nature does recognize the complexity of help required by these children. Such heavily manned clinics are luxuries which few health services can afford and, for the vast mass of children with weight problems today, they are not an available option.

Table 3.1. Advantages and disadvantages of various possible care options for overweight children

Place	Type of set-up and clinic 'leader'	Advantages	Disadvantages	General comments
Hospital	General clinic: paediatrician	Child is not necessarily stigmatized by attending paediatric clinic. Easy access to other paediatric facilities.	Unlikely to be time for full evaluation and advice. Most hospitals are unsympathetic towards spending money and clinical time for what are seen as essentially 'healthy' children. Hospital context may lead to many referrals from other clinics overemphasizing abnormality in obesity and inhibiting 'normal' obese.	The paediatric environment is helpful but hospitals are essentially 'threatening' to families and children. Staff may not be empathic to the obese. Frequent follow-up is often difficult because of pressure from other clinical work.
	Endocrine clinic: paediatric endocrinologist	Child can be investigated by specialists.	Complex investigation not necessary for most children. Specialists have insufficient time and interest to set aside for full advice.	No need for paediatric endocrinologists to be involved in routine management. Some individual paediatric endocrinologists have set up effective clinics often run by others.
	Obesity clinic: paediatrician, community paediatrician, dietician or multidisciplinary team	Focus on the needs of families and obese children in a paediatric environment. Can be a single professional or a multidisciplinary team.	Needs health workers with time and hospital management support. Dependent on enthusiastic individuals. The distance subjects have to travel can lead to poor clinic attendance.	Can be very effective but the costs of a hospital-sited clinic are considerable. Multidisciplinary teams may seem ideal but are often impractical.

Table 3.1. (cont.)

Place	Type of set-up and clinic 'leader'	Advantages	Disadvantages	General comments
	Obesity group	Advantages from children joining in activities with other children who are also overweight/obese. Multidisciplinary support and advice can be a great advantage.	Does not suit all children nor all families. Evidence suggests that with only psychological support and no input on diet children end up happier but just as overweight.	Type of group varies from clinical psychologist only to multidisciplinary team. May be difficult for children and families to have individual advice or to discuss personal issues. Difficult to arrange place and staff unless funded research project.
General practice	Routine surgery: general practitioner	Children likely to present here first. Less threatening environment than hospital. General practitioners should have good understanding of family background.	Usually insufficient time to assess and advise adequately. Frequent follow-up not very practical especially at times of year when the clinic is very busy.	Practice may have little experience in managing overweight children. Families sometimes advised inappropriately 'It's just puppy fat' or 'You can't do anything about it.' Can be a useful initiator and supporter of weight control measures advised elsewhere.
	Obesity clinic: general practitioner or practice nurse	Likely to be fairly easily accessible. Knowledge of family/social environments. Could be run by practice nurse.	Unlikely that surgeries have a set-up particularly for overweight children. Managing children with adults may not be appropriate.	Problems with sustainability of clinic when other pressures on practice time and finances. Needs suitably knowledgeable and enthusiastic members of practice.

Community	School clinic: school nurse or community paediatrician	Readily accessible for the children and in familiar environment. School staff can provide supportive back-up.	Labels children as obese to their peers. May encourage teasing and bullying. Difficult for parents to attend during working hours. Both Cochrane Reviews suggest the school is an appropriate setting for prevention but not for treatment interventions.	A specific clinic for children with weight problems seems too likely to label children negatively to their friends. Schools helpful in providing clubs offering activity, help with self-esteem or with interests which divert children's attentions from food.
	Commercial 'slimming' club: run by nutritionist or dietetic 'consultant'	These clubs often well organized with back-up literature and varied support programmes.	Most clubs designed for adults with little experience of obese children. Heavy emphasis on weight loss and adult ambience unsuitable for children. Can be expensive.	Older children may find these useful when they go with an overweight parent. Presence of overweight adults with significant co-morbidities not helpful.
	Community multifaceted project led by nutritionist, nurse, paediatrician or other interested professional	Companionship and infective enthusiasm help promote self-esteem. Multi-pronged approach to issues around the obesity can be very helpful. Short course approach focuses on targets.	Many of these projects are research activities and not yet launched into communities. Funding can be a problem. Cost-effectiveness has yet to be shown.	Potential for managing significant numbers of children within the community and the family. Positive messages from the project may be spread through the community. Needs team of professionals who can generate enthusiasm in their clients. Strong subject commitment to the scheme.

How?

The management of obesity involves a number of steps, the first and most important of which is that the obese children and their families acknowledge the need for help. Other steps follow. Thus the process of managing the obesity could be seen as the following progression:

- gain initial recognition from child and family that overweight/obesity is a problem
- find a location that will provide appropriate help for child and family
- assess the child and the severity of the problem
- recognize and investigate any underlying problems to the obesity
- treat or refer children with the complications of obesity
- develop long-term commitment to weight control from child and family
- advise on diet and eating habits
- advise on physical activity and reducing sedentariness
- advise on psychosocial problems
- encourage follow-up
- evaluate the effect of the programme on child and family
- use the findings of evaluations to improve the overall programme
- develop face-saving exit strategies for children who make no progress despite management input.

Forms of management

Individual management

Children are usually seen individually in general practice surgeries or paediatric hospital units. Facilities could be dedicated clinics or group sessions or a combination of the two. In our experience it is almost impossible to provide the right atmosphere and to focus on the weight problem and the behavioural and lifestyle issues that surround being obese if children are seen only in the usually busy, sickness-orientated environment of a surgery or general paediatric clinic. A study of a select group of general practitioners who had expressed interest in managing obese adults indicated that very few spent more than 10 minutes with each obese subject (Counterweight Project Team 2004; Laws 2004). Much longer is needed. Thus a specific obesity facility needs to be developed. If such a facility can be 'demedicalized' this could encourage attendance but inspiration may be needed for this.

Children can present with significant weight problems at any age, but many present in adolescence. Adolescents pose problems to children's hospitals whenever they require help since paediatric units are often more focused on younger age groups. Small chairs, toys and the presence of many uncontrolled youngsters are not 'cool'. Ideally facilities should provide different sessions for adolescents and for younger children. Facilities should also be comfortable both for large children and for their possibly larger parents. For example, some armless chairs in clinic and waiting rooms allow for the obese to overlap the chairs rather than be squashed into them. Some general practices are involved in the Counterweight programme (Broom and Haslam 2004; Broom et al. 2004; Counterweight Project Team 2004; McQuigg et al. 2005) for the management of adult obesity. Here trained practice nurses implement obesity management in groups, clinics or opportunistically and are supported by educational materials and backed up by weight management advisors. Evaluation is only just beginning but the support offered to practitioners by this programme would seem likely to make practices more active in the management of obesity. Similar programmes are needed for childhood weight problems. The WATCH IT programme based at the University of Leeds is one such programme still at a relatively early stage of development (Rudolf et al. 2006).

Group management

Community weight management groups, directed towards helping overweight children and their families, open up less 'medically' orientated opportunities for these children. Few such programmes for children currently exist in the UK. Private 'slimming' groups are geared towards adults. The goals and expectations of such groups together with their often middle-aged female clientele make them unsuitable for the management of obese children. In the UK there are few health service based groups for children. Evidence largely from North America indicates that groups focusing on behavioural and personality changes amongst obese children and their families have little effect unless the programmes are supported by advice on diet and activity as well (Foster et al. 2005; Savoye et al. 2005).

Multifaceted research programmes such as the MEND (Mind, Exercise, Nutrition and Do it) programme developed at the Institute of Child Health at Great Ormond Street Hospital in London seem comparatively successful (Sacher et al. 2005). The MEND programme is directed at children between 7 and 13 years old and uses techniques and goals that aim to create behavioural changes which modify energy intakes, encourage enjoyable activity, improve understanding of behavioural change and give practical help to families for diet, physical activity and family functioning. Children attend for weekly 2-hour sessions over 12 weeks. This programme is gathering momentum with support from the National Lottery, Sport England, Sainsbury's and several primary care trusts (PCTs). The outcome of intervention on this scale could be very informative. There are a number of similar programmes developing in the UK which focus on making dietary change and activity enjoyable and which encourage children to control their weight change themselves as far as practical. Many are research programmes. Translating successful research projects into programmes that are financially viable and sustainable within communities is not easy.

Residential management

Summer camps for overweight children have had a lot of publicity in the media (Gately *et al.* 2005). The camps are successful in helping children's self-esteem, improving their activity levels and to some extent reducing their weight but many families are not prepared to send their obese children away from home. The camp ambience does not suit all children. Camps are too expensive and short term to be major players in the management of child-hood obesity. Nevertheless, the lessons learned from the experiences with overweight children at these camps can be useful when planning strategies for the management of childhood overweight in other spheres.

In France very overweight children are sometimes admitted long term to units run by paediatricians (Frelut 2002). The admission may be for many months and interventions cover many aspects of the child's and the family's life. Health services in the UK are unlikely to be persuaded that such units are necessary or cost effective. For a very few children showing severe compli-cations of obesity (see Chapter 6), hospital admission for urgent weight reduction can be lifesaving.

Computer-based weight control advice

Several adult 'slimming' groups offer help and advice through computer-based services as well as, or as alternatives to, their group sessions. Advice for children through web pages is less well developed and we are a little reluctant to encourage something which leads children to the television or computer screen when this sedentary occupation is one we are recommending should decrease (see Chapter 10). Children very addicted to the internet might possibly follow guidance from a website with more enthusiasm than listening to advice from a live individual and the experience of interventionists in the USA shows this approach should be developed further. A list of useful websites is provided in Table 3.2.

Aspects common to all projects for childhood weight management

The prevalence of childhood overweight and obesity today would suggest to us that some form of multifaceted community project is going to be the only

Table 3.2. Some websites 'for children' advising on healthy lifestyle and positive self-regard

UK	www.toast-uk.org
	www.mendprogramme.org
	www.teenagehealthfreak.org
	www.lifebytes.gov.uk
Australia	www.goforyourlife.vic.gov.au
	www.completelygorgeous.com.au
	www.daa.asn.au
USA	www.cyh.com
	www.learntobehealthy.org

way to have significant impact on the large numbers of children already obese. Meanwhile the practical reality is that facilities for obese children are provided by those who are keen to help these children in whatsoever places are available for management. A variety of approaches will probably always be necessary since childhood obesity is unlikely to be solved by 'one size fits all'.

Ambience

Management must take place in an environment where children and their families feel welcome and helpers are non-judgemental. This applies to both clinicians seeing the children and clinic support staff. There should be opportunities both for parents and for children – especially adolescents – to speak with the health worker separately (Dixon-Woods *et al.* 1999). Particularly for older children, weighing, measuring and clinical examination should be carried out in an area where privacy can be respected. For young preschool and early school years overweight/obese children, advice should be directed more towards the parents than the children although the more the children feel involved and can take control the better, since they need to learn and practise weight controlling behaviours which they can continue through life.

Adolescents should be enabled to take control of the management of their weight problem much more than younger children (McPherson 2005). The role of parents, although important, should be to support the adolescent rather than to organize their weight management. It can be helpful if children and families waiting to be seen have opportunity to meet and talk with others with similar problems in a relaxed atmosphere or can be invited to join group activities involving parents and children which enhance the support and advice provided in the clinic.

Frequency of attendance

Frequent attendance for progress assessment and advice seems associated with greater success over weight control. Follow-up within two 2 weeks of initial attendance should provide support for efforts being made (before the child becomes bored with 'trying' to lose weight) and help with areas where implementing advice is proving difficult. Frequent attendances can put a strain on families who may have to travel some distance or for children at critical points in their education. There must be a balance for each family between what might be ideal and what is sustainable in their particular circumstances. We discuss reviews for these children further in Chapter 12 but the need for large numbers of follow up attendances must be incorporated into any facility for the obese.

Targets and intended outcomes?

Targets/goals for the management of overweight children must be realistic and achievable. Expectations may have to be dashed. Losing 10 kg of overweight in 2 weeks in order to look good as a bridesmaid is not realistic. But other expectations can be the opposite: 'Diets don't work. We've tried everything. Nothing can be done.' Time and careful explanation are needed to create reasonable expectations. What is feasible will depend on the child's degree of overweight, age and physical maturity, family history of overweight, previous experience over attempting weight control, duration of overweight and, most importantly, the interest and ability of child and family to implement advice.

If children are excessively overweight, particularly with adolescents nearing the end of linear growth, restoration of normal weight and normal BMI in the foreseeable future is unlikely. But any fat reduction is beneficial for health (Vanhala *et al.* 1998). The target is not necessarily to achieve normal weight. Even no weight loss but significant change in diet and improved levels of physical activity may reduce the risks of developing co-morbidities in later life (Reinehr *et al.* 2005). Setting a suitable target for a very overweight child can be difficult. No further weight gain should be one target and making recommendations for an acceptable rate of weight loss which would help the fat reduction process should be suggested. Once it is clear to what extent child and family are committed to the process and able to achieve, more specific targets may be settable. It may be better to focus interest on achieving targets based on behaviour changes which affect diet and activity rather than focus always on change in weight or fatness, the effect of which can be that the child and family are often disappointed in what they achieve despite what, to them, seems great effort (Savoye *et al.* 2005).

Some recommend that weight loss should not be an aim in the management of childhood obesity. Targets should be for children to maintain

Table 3.3. Weights of mean, borderline overweight and borderline obese BMI[a] for children with height on 80th centile for age at ages 2, 8, 12 and 16 years

	Age (years)			
	2	8	12	16
Boys				
80th centile height for age (cm)[b]	88.3	131.5	156.0	179.6
Weight for mean BMI (kg)	12.9	27.3	42.3	64.6
Weight, borderline overweight (kg)	14.4	31.8	51.5	77.1
Weight, borderline obesity (kg)	15.6	37.4	63.2	93.4
Girls				
80th centile height for age (cm)[b]	87.2	131.5	157.3	168
Weight for mean BMI (kg)	12.4	27.5	44.7	57.5
Weight, borderline overweight (kg)	13.7	31.6	53.6	68.8
Weight, borderline obesity (kg)	15.0	37.3	65.9	82.9

[a] Using IOTF cut-off points (Cole *et al.* 2000).
[b] World Health Organization (1983).

constant weight whilst they 'grow into their weight'. Yes, most children have the possibility of growing into their weight – but for some this process requires years of weight maintenance. Is it inspirational to keep weight static for 3 – or more – years (for example)? If the child is already over expected adult weight (and many attending clinics are) no weight change will result in a gradual reduction in excess BMI but accepts a certain level of adult obesity. Striving for some weight reduction, however slight, should theoretically be easier when children are still using energy in growth, and should ultimately reduce the level of adult obesity and perhaps the risk of later morbidity.

Public understanding equates treating obesity with weight loss. Education of obese children and their families needs to make it clear that static weights can indicate fat loss. However, at the same time, the aim should be for some small steady weight loss since this can provide encouragement to those who have no desire to continue attending the weight control clinic for ever. In Table 3.3 mean and borderline weights for overweight and obesity are given for relatively tall boys and girls at different ages. These give some indication of the weight losses needed to escape from the overweight category although as children are growing, the actual weight – provided it does not increase – and the target weight will draw closer.

On average, between the ages of 10 and 11, girls gain around 4.5 kg/year and boys gain slightly less (World Health Organization 1983). Because of the three-dimensional nature produced by age, growth in height and thus normally a gain in weight, predicting when a particular height will grow into

Table 3.4. Suggested maximum rates of average weight loss for management of obese children at different ages

Age group	Weight change
Under 2 years	Aim for weight gain slower than normal or weight maintenance; weight loss no more than 125 g/week
2–5 years	Weight maintenance or loss no greater than 125 g/week
5–10 years	Small weight losses helpful as targets; rates of loss no greater than 250 g/week
Girls 10–menarche	Weight loss desirable except for mildest cases; losses no more than 500 g/week
Girls post-menarche (i.e. growth slowing or ceased)	Weight loss should be targeted; losses no greater than 500 g/week
Boys >10 years	Rapid growth rates during puberty; no loss or small weight losses can be associated with useful falls in BMI; weight losses no more than 500 g/week

weight is difficult. However, a child of 10 years old who is 10 kg above the weight that creates an 'overweight' BMI will need to maintain weight stable for more than a year before BMI is likely to fall into the normal category. Children aged 10 presenting with overweight are frequently *much* more than 10 kg overweight.

What rates of weight loss should be targeted?

In Table 3.4 we provide some rather arbitrary maxima for average rates of weight loss that we feel can be achieved without producing concerning negative energy balance such that it might affect linear growth. Weight losses averaging more than these over a couple of weeks should stimulate review of how they are being achieved. Should a more relaxed attitude to weight control be recommended? There is a fine balance between achieving effective management and creating what could be too great an energy deficit. High weight losses achieved because of greatly increased physical activity could be more acceptable than those achieved by predominantly very strict control of energy intakes. However, weight losses are often relatively high between initial appointment and first follow-up since the reduced carbohydrate intakes that may accompany changes to more organized eating can be associated with loss of body water leading to noticeable weight loss unrelated to fat loss. This is an initial drop only.

Targets for behavioural and weight changes will probably need revising when reviewing children's achievements between attendances. Whatever targets are set, all weight loss or fall in BMI centile position should be applauded and encouraged as should all evidence of effort put into changing to more weight controlling lifestyles.

Targets for infants and toddlers

Table 3.3 shows how the weight differences between normal, overweight and obese categories are smaller for young children (who have also had less time to get very overweight) than for older children. In the very young, rates of growth are fast (although they slow dramatically over the first 6 months of life). Weight gains slower than expected for age can be associated with quite rapid falls in BMI for age. As infants mature and begin to weight bear there is a period of physiological slimming and fall in %BF (see Chapter 2) which can work to the advantage of very young children whose parents are keen to bring weight under control. A 'sensible' diet and the provisions of opportunities for young children to be as active as possible (see Chapters 9 and 10) may be all that is needed to restore normal weight and BMI. Even so, if young children are very overweight, low levels of weight loss can be targets but the situation needs supervision by those experienced in monitoring the growth of these young people.

Recommendations

- There is no single answer to what should be provided as the ideal set-up for the management of obesity and overweight in children. The varied personalities and family expectations of obese children will probably always necessitate a variety of opportunities for those seeking help. Set-ups that provide experiences which involve children and families in positive personality development, nutrition education, improved eating habits and activity in enjoyable surroundings seem likely to be more effective than 'group' or clinic set-ups which only suggest this through verbal advice.
- Facilities of any kind, with input from professionals who have time to advise and to show enthusiasm for overweight/obese children, are currently desperately needed.
- The targets set for overweight/obese children must be realistic. They should not raise unachievable expectations but should inspire families that weight control is possible.
- Some time limit on achieving a target should be set so management does not drag on ineffectively and endlessly. Teaching child and family that any reduction in fat and/or improved cardiorespiratory function is beneficial for long-term health should encourage even the most obese to make some effort to change their lifestyles (see Chapter 8).

4

How do we approach the overweight/obese child and family?

Families seek advice on their children's weight problems for various reasons. Some children are concerned about their weight and are openly asking for help. Some children are brought by concerned parents but the children, because they are very young or for other reasons, are themselves unconcerned by their overweight. Some parents and children come to the clinic but deny weight is a problem, and the parents are not prepared to talk about the problem in front of their children or pretend they have no concerns about their children's weights. They attend because others – friends, relatives or the school – have told them they 'must do something about the weight'. Initial approaches to overweight children and their families need to bear in mind these different presentations. Health care practitioners (HCPs) should avoid seeming to criticize parents or to refer automatically to the children as obese since some families are very sensitive to any mention of overweight and, even more, of obesity. Nevertheless, HCPs need to help families develop realistic understanding of the children's overweight and of the need for action.

Once the subject of the child's weight has been broached, first contact with overweight children and their families should focus on the families' expectations from the attendance (Wardle *et al.* 1995). For some, modifying over-ambitious ideas about what management of overweight can achieve is important. For others, gaining the confidence of families who may have very low self-esteem and no faith in their ability to make effective change is fundamental to implementing any management. The difficulties this latter group of families have in accepting their children are significantly overweight and that changes are needed relate in part to the negative, but widely held, societal attitudes about obesity. Such attitudes are common even amongst HCPs and can be encompassed by the following views:

- excessive weight is self-inflicted due to over-indulgence and lack of will-power
- excessive weight is a lifestyle rather than a medical issue

- excessive weight is, in the case of children, a failing of parental responsibility.

These views do not take into account the recent social and environmental changes which encourage weight gain. Many of these changes are outside the control of the children or parents. Thus holding parents responsible for their children's weight is too simplistic, is unhelpful in developing management strategies and can act as a barrier to working with the family (Edmunds 2005).

The parents' perspective

Most parents have some idea of the relative size of their children because clothes are sold in age sizes. Parents of overweight children are often less adept at judging overweight in their children, particularly in boys, compared with parents of normal weight children. They may not be convinced by the age sizes nor appreciate the consequences of their children being outsize, particularly if there is a history of overweight in the family. Also parents may not perceive health risks in the same way that health professionals do in that risks can have positive connotations (exciting or exploratory) as well as negative ones (dangerous or harmful).

Parents can be grouped according to their perspective on the child's overweight into:

- those who recognize the problem and have tried self-help approaches to control weight which have not been effective and so seek further advice
- those who are aware of the problem but are still coming to terms with the need for action
- those who want support for the self-help approaches they have initiated
- those who are not aware of the significance of their child's excessive weight but are ready to accept advice and help
- those who are aware their child is overweight but see this as 'inevitable', 'their family's size', 'not a subject for discussion', or 'not a matter for interference from outside the family'.

Sensitivity, tact and uncritical approaches are needed to work with these different views.

What rouses parental concerns about children's weights?

Parents go through processes of realization and action (Figure 4.1). Asking for help is often precipitated by their child suffering a bullying incident. Parents then gauge the seriousness of the problem by monitoring their children's social competences. If their children have plenty of friends, parents are usually less concerned than when children are isolated and unsupported

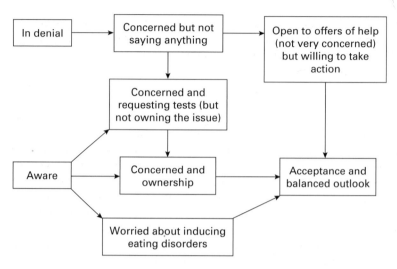

Figure 4.1 Processes that parents may go through in recognizing their child's weight problem.

by peers (Jain *et al.* 2001). A number of children are referred under pressure from their schools because they are obese and failing educationally or having difficulty making peer relationships at school. Schools may suggest that reducing the overweight will improve educational progress but, in our experience, these children often have learning difficulties. These lead to isolation from peers and that causes, rather than is caused by, the obesity.

When asked how they would like to be treated by HCPs, parents of overweight and obese children make a number of relevant points. They want HCPs to show they understand how complicated it can be bringing up an overweight child. Coping with everyday family management and acting to control their children's weights challenge family dynamics and may have repercussions beyond the immediate family. Parents – and children – want their views to be heard. They do not want formulaic responses but information they can understand together with feedback on action and progress.

How HCPs and parents involve themselves in managing weight problems depends on the age and maturity of children. With preschool children parents have control over most aspects of their children's lives and particularly over what and when the children eat and how much opportunity they have for vigorous exercise. As children grow older these controls diminish. By adolescence the parents are still in the position of responsibility, supporting and insisting on some carefully selected rules of behaviour but the independence, self-determination and decision-making of the adolescent are paramount in many areas that concern weight. Parents and HCPs must recognize this if their advice is to be heeded at all. Specific age-related approaches to weight management are discussed further later. Here we deal with more generic approaches to controlling overweight.

What do parents want to know?

When parents reach the point where they want to talk to an outsider about their child's weight, the following are likely to be uppermost in their minds:

- They want to discuss their child's overweight without the child being present. The child may not be aware of the weight problems and the parents may not want to raise such concerns, especially in front of HCPs they have not met before. Or the child may be very sensitive about the problem and parents may wish to hide their own concern from their child.
- Mothers particularly have fears of inducing an 'eating disorder'/'slimmer's disease' if any action is taken to control weight gain. These fears may stifle all consideration of changing dietary behaviours.
- Parents may be concerned about medical reasons for the overweight and want investigation and reassurance.

Whatever their concerns, parents deserve to be heard, to have their requests taken seriously and to be treated empathetically regardless of whether they themselves are overweight or not. Around 80% of all communication is non-verbal. Posture, facial expressions and tone of voice convey more meaning than words. Negative and/or uneasy feelings are likely to be sensed by parents and their children and construed as criticism or disapproval. Negative reactions create defensive responses, offence and/or resentment.

Research looking at 'communicating sad, bad and difficult news' (Fallowfield and Jenkins 2004) suggests that effective communication is enhanced by practitioners showing concern rather than professional detachment, appearing confident but caring, having written information available and allowing families time for questions.

So, when parents of the obese or overweight ask for help:

- React sympathetically, genuinely and positively.
- Listen to their concerns and offer investigation as appropriate.
- Ask parents and children for their views on why there is overweight.
- Probe gently for other events in the background which may be driving or exacerbating the weight gain (e.g. grief, bullying, parental disagreement over child management).
- Be ready to refer children and families to professionals with other skills. These families may need help from education psychologists, child guidance clinics, social services, debt management advisors, grief counsellors or other counsellors.
- Recognize that if there are family problems, behaviour change is likely to be much harder to address.

Table 4.1. Points about weight control to be made to families of overweight children

Weight control –
- is not easy
- is not quick
- is not something for the child to manage alone
- is something that should not be allowed to develop into a family battleground (especially important when dealing with adolescents)
- is something that must be potentially sustainable for each individual child and family
- is something in which the whole family should have constructive involvement
- is something where parents, friends and relatives should show consistency
- is something where parents and children should discuss behavioural changes together
- is something on which children should be allowed, as appropriate to their age and development, to make decisions about what they will or will not do
- is something which can have beneficial effects for health and well-being for all even if ultimate goals for weight control are not reached

- Do not assume asking for help means that parents and children are at ease discussing all their problems.
- Do not assume asking for help means that parents or children will necessarily implement any advice given.
- If parents or children do not seem to want to discuss issues outside their weight problem and how to control this, there is no value in pushing for revelation of underlying issues. Under duress, children and families are likely to provide socially desirable but not necessarily honest answers.

At some point the interview has to move to constructive planning for weight management. More than kind words are needed if children with persistent weight problems and their families are to implement changes which address reducing their excess fat. What action should be advised is put forward in subsequent chapters. Table 4.1 lists general points that could be appropriate introduction to the guidance about weight management for most families.

Some parents need a lot of convincing that they, or their children, can control their weight problem. This may be because of previous failure to control weight either in themselves or in their children. Setting a stricter weight control regime for a longer period than previously experienced may be what is needed to be effective. Thus, whilst we usually suggest small incremental changes for the management of overweight, when developing a weight control programme for 'failed' dieters, a short period of a disciplined regime such as exclusion of all high energy snack products may effect weight loss and show child and family that 'dieting' can work. This may provide the evidence needed to make child and family take long-term interest in active weight management.

Some parents are daunted by the prospect of trying to control their child's weight through changes in diet and activity ('Isn't there a pill you can give?'). They feel they have neither the time nor the resources (internal and external) to cope, particularly if they have had difficulty managing their own weight. They need to be reassured that, whatever the parental size or family situation, parents are effective agents of change for the family (Summerbell *et al.* 2003). Supporting the parents to enable them to change lifestyle behaviours is crucially dependent on good relationships between families and HCPs, whether general practitioners (GPs), paediatricians, dietitians, practice nurses or others.

How to approach the children

We have discussed gaining understanding from the parents but what about the children? Too often parents and children do not present a unified front over how seriously they view the weight problem and the need to take action. Often this is because parents are anxious to implement weight control activities and the children appear to have neither concern about their weight nor interest in taking any action. Sometimes, although this may be only subtly hinted, the children are trying to implement weight controlling guidance but receive inadequate support from one or both parents. Sometimes seeming indifference is the child's way of manipulating parents. In adolescence, this can be a very effective way of demonstrating independence and own will.

When children express no interest in participating in any attempts at weight control it may be best to leave discussion about implementing change to the parents at home rather than seeming to side with parental authority. Sometimes it may be helpful to ask these children either to say or to write down what they perceive as the advantages and disadvantages of being overweight, of taking action over their weight and of the difficulties they experience or anticipate when considering weight control. This can be revealing both regarding children's perceptions of their weight problem and regarding some of the issues behind their persistent obesity. Contrary to much public opinion many obese children are happy, well integrated and not bothered about their obesity. However getting the children to try looking objectively at their condition can both give the advisors some points with which to discuss positive solutions and help the children focus more on their perceptions so they realize benefits should accrue if they could only control their weight a little (Figure 4.2).

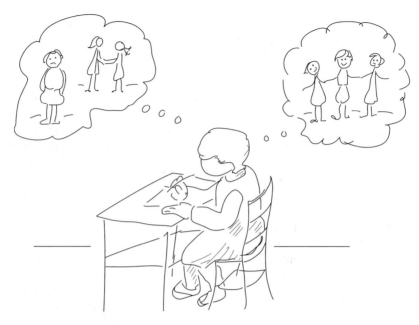

Figure 4.2 Some children may be able to express their thoughts better through writing than talking.

Giving advice

Whilst some families expect to be handed a diet sheet and strict instructions on what to do to control their children's weight, the complexity surrounding the development of obesity and the individuality of families makes it advisable to work with the child and family on developing a 'personalized' management policy. Specific lifestyle changes recommended, especially those involving dietary changes, can be listed but the list should be drawn up in the clinic together with each subject child and family. Peterson (2005) has drawn attention to the need to use solution-building interview questions rather than problem-solving questions when trying to help overweight children and their families develop a management plan for themselves. Clinics dedicated to obesity management may wish to develop their own framework advice sheets to which individualized recommendations can be added. We discuss specific issues on management in subsequent chapters but make some general points here.

Programmes for weight management which cause rapid and dramatic changes in weight generally have little long-term sustainability. Moreover, and this is particularly important in relation to children since they are growing and depositing lean tissue, the weight lost, if it is lost quickly on a 'crash' diet, may contain unnecessary loss of lean tissue. Since it is difficult to implement any lifestyle change for the families of overweight children, it would seem likely to be more difficult to make many substantial changes. Thus programmes should include a few achievable changes in the first instance (Peterson 2005). Support from other family members who may have to endure a lot of interference in their own lifestyles is also likely to be less than with more modest changes. If small changes can be implemented, and particularly if changes begin to improve the children's well-being or weight status, families may grow in confidence over their ability to make changes and be more prepared to take on subsequent step-by-step change.

Thus, as generalizations, we recommend that lifestyle strategies to enable weight control should include:

- involving child and adolescent as much as appropriate for age and development
- ensuring that parents recognize their own role in the initiation and implementation of family change and family support for the child
- suggesting small but incremental changes appropriate to the child and family's lifestyle, starting with a few changes and building on these
- taking a long-term perspective to management but having some endpoint even if the endpoint needs later re-evaluation for long-term goals. (Without some endpoint, management can drag on interminably with unclear objectives.)

Difficult age groups

Preschool children

Most parents of preschool children have had some recent contact with their health visitors or practice nurses. They are used to having their children weighed and measured. They may however be very sensitive to any comment about their children's weight – whether the suggestion is that the weight gain is inadequate or too great. Plotting weights and lengths on growth charts and showing progress to parents can be useful not only in opening the way for conversations about weight, but also for demonstrating where children are in relation to population norms. Mothers and health visitors view this approach as an appropriate way to introduce the subject of children's weights (Edmunds *et al.* 2007). It may then be possible to detect how receptive mothers (usually mothers) are likely to be to discussing their children's weights. The result of this will determine whether advice is initiated then or whether the mother goes off to consider the matter and discuss it with her partner. Any resistance to the idea that the child is overweight probably means the parents are not yet ready to embark on what may be perceived as socially stigmatizing discussions. There is little point in pushing a conversation with a parent who is not listening.

Despite the above, the action of advisors must be tempered by assessment of the extent of children's problems (if any other than overweight). Young children who are very overweight and have unremitting excessive weight gain, or who have other problems such as slow development, need investigation for underlying contributing medical conditions (see Chapter 5). Significant concern should be indicated confidentially and delicately (as should happen with any health worker–client discussion) when possible medical complications are being raised. The need for further assessment should be stressed. Large, active, normally responsive young children who are overweight but not increasingly so are likely to excite less immediate concern. Their parents should be allowed time to decide what action they want to take to further weight management.

If mothers perceive their children to be happy, healthy and with plenty of friends, they tend not to worry about them regardless of the size they are. Bringing up the subject of overweight is 'like walking on egg shells'.

Adolescents

Patton and Viner (2007) draw attention to the neurodevelopment that continues through adolescence into adulthood and the biological gap this produces between physical maturity and emotional and behavioural maturity. Refining self-control and judgement may continue long after adolescence has passed. Thus, around the age of puberty, children enhance their decision-making abilities. They have usually been told what, how and when to do things by parents, teachers and other adults most of their lives and are now determined to make decisions for themselves. This is a natural and necessary part of growing up and key to establishing personal independence. However, if adolescents make 'wrong' decisions or decisions that are different from significant others, they soon learn that this:
- creates separation very effectively
- develops their independence and freedom
- gives them opportunity to exercise power over their parents (and other adults).

Where families have clear, well-established and fair boundaries to behaviour, less energy is spent by the adolescents challenging these boundaries. Additionally, parents in more functional families are likely to expand the boundaries as their children grow up. Dramatic adolescent behaviours are then not necessary for the development of a growing sense of being one's own person. Where there is a disorganized lifestyle with no consistent parenting, children and adolescents have difficulty learning acceptable behaviours. To make a sweeping generalization, the more dysfunctional the family, the more traumatic life with an adolescent is likely to be.

Working with adolescents can be difficult as HCPs may try to adopt 'parental' roles. One approach is to try to see the world from the young person's perspective whilst still remaining impartial. Adolescents no longer want to be ordered around and yet are still in the process of learning that making their own decisions carries responsibility. In our experience, the following points may help working with adolescents:

- Try to give adolescents the opportunity to be seen on their own. They may have issues that they feel uncomfortable discussing in front of parents.
- If parents and adolescents are only seen jointly, direct questions and responses primarily at the adolescents rather than the parents – although making sure parents are included in the discussion. The aim is to let adolescents speak for themselves with parents in supporting roles. The extent to which this happens will depend on the age and confidence of the adolescents involved. A strongly adolescent-centred approach may not be appropriate for those with learning difficulties or emotional immaturity.
- Create the notion for the adolescents that making their own decisions is fine but they must take responsibility for these decisions. For example if they feel it is important for social reasons that they eat in a fast food restaurant, then they need to acknowledge that their weight will be more difficult/impossible to control if they continue to do this. They may, or may not, be able to compensate by eating less when there is no social imperative or by being more active – they have to choose whether they will run this risk.
- Remember adolescents are much more likely to be cooperative if they are not challenged, particularly in front of their parents. Both parties may find such a challenge embarrassing and demeaning.
- Recognize that it may be necessary to point out unintentionally unhelpful comments made by parents. This should not be done in front of the adolescents. 'I told you so' type comments or derogatory remarks about adolescents' fledgling efforts to take action act to maintain barriers which may be preventing the young people making positive changes to their lives. They may even worsen already difficult situations.
- Acknowledge that changing behaviours is as difficult for adolescents as it is for adults but adolescents have all the added baggage of establishing their independence and dealing with the physical demands of growth. Trying to motivate them with thoughts of short-term benefits such as being able to wear more fashionable clothes or finding it easier to be active with their peers is more effective than offering the prospect of long-term health benefits which provide little incentive even to overweight adults. Motivating discussions take time.
- Recognize that sometimes adolescents perceive their lives as already too complicated for them to work at weight control. Where there is no

effective change in the overweight and particularly if attempts to encourage weight control are only leading to unproductive confrontations between adolescents and their parents, it is wise to accept with the adolescent that the time for weight control is not now and to advise parents appropriately.

Working with adolescents is about respecting them as individuals and supporting them in their decision-making so they learn to make decisions that are beneficial in the long run. These are transferable skills although our particular focus is on developing decisions about healthy eating, physical activity and emotional well-being.

Often young people find it easier to accept advice from adults outside the family as they have no emotional complications with them and much less to fight against. Nevertheless, parents still have an important role to play. They need to be supportive to their adolescents who are trying to control over-weight. They should avoid being judgemental or critical. Support often means being prepared to listen to their adolescent child even if the way in which things are expressed are not conducive to harmony. Despite adoles-cents' growing independence, they are likely to be housed and financially supported by parents. Acceptable behaviours or rules for very specific and necessary issues need to be agreed with consultation between parents and the young person. If any retribution for breaking the rules is deemed necessary this should be decided with the adolescent at the time the rules are developed rather than when they are broken. Keeping to the rules should be praised and perhaps rewarded, but not with food.

Those not interested

Some parents (and their children) will not acknowledge a weight problem let alone do anything to address weight management. These individuals 'clam up' at any mention of children's weight or related subjects. For those children or families who clearly have no interest in taking action to control over-weight, we recommend they are pleasantly and politely told no further follow-ups will be arranged but that, should they have a change of heart, 'The door of the clinic will still be open.' Obesity is difficult enough to treat in those willing to be treated without filling sessions with those who are not interested in acting or those for whom trying to control weight gain is imposing significant friction between child and parents.

Recommendations

- There are neither simple recipes nor phraseologies for approaching the issue of weight management with parents and/or children if they themselves have not raised the subject. Experience of how the family has responded to similar interventions in the past, the relationship between HCP and the family or child built up over previous contacts, and the responsiveness of members of the family on the day of presentation, all affect how any communication is interpreted. If broaching the topic is met with indifference, further discussion to encourage engagement may have to wait for a future occasion.

- If parents react to suggestions of overweight in their child with defensive responses (some parents take any criticism of their child as a slight on their child-rearing skills) it may help to explain that having an overweight child is not necessarily their fault. The child does not necessarily eat more nor exercise less than others but has needs in these areas which differ from those of normal weight peers.

- If all efforts from HCPs fail to achieve any commitment from child or family, there is little point in continuing to try to engage with the family since this may damage any positive relationship that has developed. There may be other opportunities to discuss weight management in the future or the family may return having altered their views after discussion with friends and family at home.

- Parents who raise the subject of overweight in their child without prompting may have recognized their child has a problem and may have been attempting home management unsuccessfully. They are likely to want to discuss their efforts and concerns. They are probably aware of messages about healthy eating and of the advertised benefits of activity but may be less aware of how portion sizes can be relevant to overweight or of the role played by sweetened drinks in much overweight, or they may not have recognized the relevance of sedentariness in the development of overweight.

- Identifying gaps in knowledge can be a useful first step before offering any specific guidance on weight control. Also, there may be other factors underlying the development of overweight in the child, such as parenting or family difficulties, grief and other psychological stresses. It may be necessary to address these before the family feels capable of tackling weight management.

5

The clinical assessment: what are the special points?

Most children presenting to the community with overweight or obesity have no recognizable medical condition contributing to their problem. Very rarely obesity presents as part of a specific syndrome or its development has been facilitated by an underlying medical problem. Parents sometimes attribute their child's obesity to 'the glands', a conviction which may seem to offer hope of a quick solution rather than the prospect of lifestyle changes and long-term weight monitoring. To reassure these parents and to exclude obesity syndromes all children presenting with overweight/obesity should have thorough paediatric clinical assessment.

Clinical assessment is also important to evaluate the effects of the obesity on health. Many conditions previously thought complications for long-term adult obesity only are now diagnosed in adolescents and even in much younger obese children. The first line of management for such conditions is usually reducing the excessive fatness but being made aware of developing co-morbidities may help commit some families to action over weight control. Even without the severe co-morbidities, overweight children can have orthopaedic, skin and respiratory problems exacerbated by obesity. We discuss co-morbidities briefly in Chapter 6 but any initial clinical examination must bear these potential problems in mind since they may require referral to specialist services.

Looking for underlying pathology

It is unusual for children with specific syndromes contributing to their obesity to present with obesity as the main clinical problem. The exceptions to this are children with the genetically determined leptin disorders. These children present with dramatic, uncontrollable, obesity from early life and may have affected siblings (Farooqui and O'Rahilly 2000). For most other syndromic obesity the weight problem is one clinical feature amongst more concerning clinical problems. The obesity itself may be relatively mild.

Table 5.1 lists the most likely underlying causes associated with obesity. Several of these conditions have clinical features in common. Thus some points in history and examination should alert health workers to the likelihood of an underlying clinical problem. These points include:

- Intractable severe obesity developing from birth onwards
- Progressive obesity from the first years of life
- No family history of obesity
- Short stature, especially if disproportionate growth
- Delayed puberty
- Early puberty or early adrenarche (accelerated growth and physical maturation without gonadal development) especially if associated with relatively short stature
- Clinical abnormalities:
    Musculo-skeletal abnormalities especially:
    - scoliosis
    - finger/toe abnormalities
    - dysmorphic facies
    - muscular weakness and hypotonia
    Retinitis pigmentosa
    Marked squint
- Developmental delay and learning difficulties
- Severe behavioural problems especially uncontrolled eating
- Significant psycho-emotional problems.

Pre-pubertal obese children without an underlying predisposing condition are commonly above average stature. Certain medical conditions associated with abnormally short stature (e.g. growth hormone deficiency) encourage the development of overweight. Children who are obese and below the 10th centile height for age but not concerningly short may have an obesity associated syndrome (such as Prader–Willi syndrome: PWS) where growth is less than optimal although not necessarily outside the 'normal' range. In this respect, assessment of a child's growth in relation to that expected from parental stature is relevant since the significance of, for example, a height between the 10th and 25th centile for age in a child with both parents above the 75th centile is not the same as that for a child of the same age and heaviness but with both parents on the 10th centile. As with so many other things in paediatrics, puberty complicates this picture and the relative tall stature of young overweight children is often less marked in adolescence as some obese have early puberty and end up with below average stature.

Developmental delay, major behavioural problems and poor school progress are other features which should alert health workers to the possibility of underlying conditions. These problems can be misinterpreted.

Table 5.1. Conditions that may lead to obesity or have obesity as a cardinal clinical sign

Type of condition	Specific condition	Features	Cardinal clinical features	Action if condition suspected
Genetic conditions with Mendelian inheritance	E.g. single gene disorders of leptin metabolism (usually autosomal recessive inheritance)	Very rare Gross unremitting obesity from early life	Family history of gross early-onset obesity Severe obesity from a very early age Normal or advanced linear growth	Referral to paediatric or genetic clinic
Inherited syndromes with obesity as only part of the abnormalities	Multisystem disorders with tendency to obesity, e.g. Bardet–Biedl syndrome; Alstrom syndrome; Carpenter syndrome	Obesity may not develop until post infancy; often associated short stature; may be various other congenital abnormalities; low IQ quite common concomitant condition	Short stature Psychodevelopmental delay Associated clinical abnormalities May be family history	Referral to paediatric/child development clinic for overall assessment Advice about weight control to parents when diagnosis made, even if obesity not yet present
Chromosomal disorders	E.g. Down syndrome (trisomy 21) Prader–Willi syndrome (PWS)	Psychodevelopmental problems and associated abnormalities may be more concerning than obesity initially Obesity can be gross and associated with type 2 diabetes in PWS in later childhood	May be early feeding difficulties and failure to thrive Classical clinical features involving facies, hands, hypotonia, developmental delay	If diagnosis not already made, paediatric assessment for associated severe problems Will need educational support Advise parents on diet and activity from time of diagnosis Down syndrome has high prevalence of autoimmune thyroiditis: check thyroid function

Endocrine problems	Hypothyroidism, Cushing syndrome, growth hormone deficiency	Short stature often more noticeable than obesity	Short stature developing in childhood rather than as a feature from birth. May be specific facies	Thyroid function tests. Random or fasting cortisol as screening. Refer for paediatric endocrine assessment
Central nervous system abnormalities	Craniopharyngioma. Hydrocephalus. Post encephalitis. Post cerebral irradiation. Hypotonic cerebral palsy	May be history of past central nervous system damage. Often hormonal problems emanating from hypothalamic damage	Short stature; pubertal delay; signs of raised intracranial pressure; cranial nerve palsies. Deficiencies of growth, thyroid and sex hormones	Endocrinological assessment. Check visual fields and lateral skull X-ray for calcification if craniopharyngioma suspected. CT or MRI scans may be indicated
Problems with mobility	Duchenne muscular dystrophy	In early stages of condition children often overfat although may not be overweight if much muscle wasting; may lose weight in later stages of disease	Weakness, gradual loss of weight bearing activity; sex linked recessive condition so most cases boys; often mild developmental delay	Referral to paediatric clinic if diagnosis suspected. Dietetic advice may help children and families who may 'spoil' children because of their miserable condition
	Spina bifida	Problems associated with low IQ due to hydrocephalus may contribute to tendency to obesity	Some reduced mobility due to spina bifida; hydrocephalus; may be endocrine problems arising from hypothalamic damage so may show some of the signs of endocrine problems discussed above	Encourage families to maintain as much mobility as possible despite the effort required. Advise on diet from infancy onwards. The children are likely to be attending a number of paediatric clinics already

Table 5.1. (*cont.*)

Type of condition	Specific condition	Features	Cardinal clinical features	Action if condition suspected
Bone disorders	Primary growth disorders (e.g. achondroplasia) may expend little energy in growth. Obesity rarely gross	Short stature and bony abnormalities may be obvious	Gross short stature. Disproportionate growth in many cases with short limbs and perhaps unusual facies	Obesity is not inevitable if children are active and well integrated into their community. Families should be advised on diet and activity from diagnosis
Drug treatment	Steroids	History of treatment with steroids on very regular and high dose basis. Occasionally occurs with overuse of steroid inhalers for asthma. Less likely if intermittent treatment with evening doses and lower doses	Mooning of facies; truncal obesity; purplish striae; hirsutes	Advise families on potential consequences of steroid treatment and importance of using steroids only as instructed
	Sodium valproate	History of treatment for epilepsy	Weight gain usually relates to onset of treatment	Advise families of risk of overweight on initiating therapy and suggest dietary supervision and increased exercise (if practical for affected child)

Children may be referred for obesity management because of poor school progress. Obesity is blamed for the poor self-esteem and bullying. This can be the case. Yet, in our experience, a significant number of obese children referred for these reasons are children for whom learning difficulties are actually the primary problem. Problems coping with school and consequent social isolation from peers contribute to the development of overweight/ obesity rather than the other way round. These children may or may not have specific underlying syndromes but they need psychodevelopmental and educational assessment and support as much as advice on managing their weight.

Clinical examination

Overweight and obese children (and adults) risk receiving second-rate medical assessment and treatment. Obesity can be viewed negatively by clinicians and may be dealt with somewhat peremptorily. For these reasons, whenever practical, facilities for the overweight/obese should be run by those committed and interested in caring for those with weight problems. Even when those clinically assessing the subject are dedicated and enthusiastic, practical problems make it difficult to perform first-rate clinical assessments on the very obese.

- Overweight/obese children are frequently very embarrassed by their fatness and reluctant to undress sufficiently for thorough clinical examination. A sensitive approach is needed and full clinical examination may have to wait until clinician and child and family have established a sympathetic rapport.
- Children may take a long time to undress because of the physical difficulties and embarrassment associated with their large size. This can lead to the examiner becoming impatient and performing clinical assessment under less than ideal circumstances.
- The examining clinician may have difficulty eliciting 'clinical signs' obscured by excess fat.
- Not all clinical apparatuses (e.g. weighing scales, sphygmomanometer cuffs) are geared for use with the grossly obese (see later).
- Childhood measurement 'norms' (e.g. blood pressure: BP) are often related to the child's age. Obese children are not only overweight but commonly above average stature. Findings should probably be related to build and physical maturity rather than age.
- Interpreting biochemical data in the very obese is not straightforward. Should results be related to age of the child, total weight of the child, lean body mass, 'bone age' or ...? There is no consensus.

Tables 5.2 and 5.3 list points in clinical history and examination which require particular thought when assessing obese children. As suggested above,

Table 5.2. Points for taking clinical history from an obese child

Normal clinical history including:
Child's history:
  Birth weight
  Age when obesity first noticed
  History of development of obesity, i.e. has it gradually increased or suddenly
    exacerbated?
  History of previous attempts at weight control
  Pubertal history/age at menarche if relevant age and sex
  Respiratory difficulties: snoring, sleep apnoea
  Difficulties with physical activity
  Behavioural problems especially temper tantrums, manipulation, obsessive
    compulsive features, food seeking behaviours
  Difficulties at school: cognitive and learning problems, teasing/bullying
  Child's perception of the problem of obesity
  Detailed dietary and physical activity histories (see Chapters 9 and 10)
Family history:
  Parental weights and heights
  History of obesity in family
  History of thyroid, adrenal, other hormonal problems in family
  History of diabetes (types 1 and 2); hypertension; hyperlipidaemia; early death in
    family

the clinical assessment may not be easy. The measurement and evaluation of BP can be a particular problem. What size cuff should be used on a fat arm? Systolic and diastolic BP centiles for British children have recently been published (Jackson *et al.* 2007). However these centiles still do not really indicate what is the range of normality in BP values at the different ages. These points matter since hypertension is a frequent co-morbidity of obesity in both childhood and adult life.

Measuring and interpreting blood pressure in the overweight

Various points should be observed when measuring BP in obese children (Beevers *et al.* 2001).

- Explain procedure to child/carer in a way that encourages confidence and relaxation.
- Make sure the child is resting in a sitting position with the elbow slightly flexed and supported at heart level or the child is held in this position in the carer's arms.
- Use the right arm.
- Remove any tight clothing around the upper arm.

Table 5.3. Clinical examination of the obese child[a]

Anthropometry:	
Weight and height	Calculate BMI and mark on age/sex related centile charts[b]
Waist circumference	Plot on age/sex related centile charts[c]
(Skinfold thicknesses	Plot on age/sex related centile charts[d])

General examination including looking carefully for:

Abnormal features	Suggestive of hypothyroidism
	Suggestive of hypercortisolism
	Suggestive of Prader–Willi syndrome (see Table 5.6)
	Suggesting other 'obesity syndrome'
Skin problems	Intertrigo
	Acanthosis nigra
	Signs of self-mutilitation
	Excessive purplish striae
Orthopaedic problems:	Genu valgum
	Any suggestion of hip problems
	Other congenital bony abnormality
Other:	Blood pressure (see Tables 5.4 and 5.5)
	Cardiorespiratory problems
	Hepatomegaly

Behaviour
Intellectual ability
Emotional stability

[a] This examination includes assessing both for underlying pathology and co-morbidities of obesity.
[b] Harlow Printing Company (2007).
[c] Child Growth Foundation (2007).
[d] The British skinfold for age centile charts are very out of date: Tanner and Whitehouse (1975).

- Ensure the inflatable sphygmomanometer bladder encompasses at least 80% but no more than 100% of the upper arm circumference (see Table 5.4).
- Choose a cuff with depth about one-third the length of the upper arm (see Table 5.4).
- Place the cuff over the brachial artery leaving room below for the stethoscope (if manual reading) to be applied to the brachial artery just above the elbow.
- Palpate the pulse when first deflating the cuff so that very high systolic endpoints are not missed by a period of silence between systolic and diastolic sounds. Sounds can be difficult to hear with young children and it may only be possible to obtain a palpated systolic measurement.

Table 5.4. Size of inflatable bladder on sphygmomanometer cuff for children

Maximum arm circumference for this cuff (cm)	Cuff bladder width (cm)	Cuff bladder length (cm)
17	4	13
26	10	18
33	12	26
50	12	40
53	20	42

Source: British Hypertension Society: //www.bhsoc.org.

- Take the first appearance of sounds and the disappearance of sounds as the systolic and diastolic points. Occasionally sounds can be heard all the way down in which case choose the muffling of sounds (Korotkoff IV) as the diastolic point (and make a note that this endpoint has been used).
- Evaluate systolic and diastolic recordings against norms for age (and perhaps BMI status) (Tables 5.5 and 5.6).

Table 5.5. Height adjusted mean systolic (standard deviation) pressures of UK children and young people aged 5–12 years on middle and upper quintiles of BMI at different ages

Age	BMI quintile: boys		BMI quintile: girls	
	Middle	Upper	Middle	Upper
5–6	105 (0.7)	107 (0.8)	106 (0.7)	106 (0.9)
7–9	107 (0.6)	108 (0.7)	109 (0.6)	111 (0.7)
10–12	111 (0.6)	114 (0.7)	113 (0.6)	117 (0.7)
13–15	119 (0.7)	125 (0.7)	117 (0.7)	123 (0.8)
16–19	128 (1.0)	134 (0.9)	119 (0.8)	121 (0.4)

Source: McMunn *et al.* (2004).

Mean systolic BP rises with increasing age and height (McMunn *et al.* 2004). Children tall for age have mean systolic BP higher than mean values for those of the same age and shorter stature. The trend holds true for systolic BP and weight for age as well. This makes interpretation of findings in overweight and obese children uncertain but the differences attributable to build in children of the same age are quite small. Significant hypertension is not easily overlooked provided BP is measured.

Table 5.6. Mean (standard deviation) systolic blood pressure for middle and tallest tertile English children aged 5–19 years

Age	Height tertile: boys		Height tertile: girls	
	Middle	Tallest	Middle	Tallest
5	106 (0.7)	105 (0.8)	104 (0.7)	105 (0.9)
7	105 (0.6)	108 (0.7)	106 (0.8)	109 (0.8)
9	109 (0.8)	111 (0.7)	109 (0.8)	113 (0.9)
11	110 (0.7)	114 (0.8)	115 (0.9)	116 (0.9)
13	116 (0.9)	122 (0.9)	117 (0.9)	118 (0.8)
15	123 (0.8)	124 (0.8)	118 (1.0)	119 (0.9)
17	129 (1.5)	127 (1.4)	121 (1.2)	121 (1.1)
19	128 (1.3)	131 (1.3)	121 (1.3)	122 (1.3)

Source: McMunn *et al.* (2004).

Obesity syndromes

We shall not describe all the conditions listed in Table 5.1 (which is by no means a complete list) since the vast majority are uncommon and in our experience rarely present with obesity as the primary problem. The list of inherited syndromes which, for example, may be associated with obesity is by no means complete. In practice many children with obesity syndromes are referred for management of their obesity from paediatric centres where their primary problems are already being followed. Prader–Willi syndrome includes many severe abnormalities other than obesity. It is a relatively common problem and occasionally a child with PWS presents with obesity without a specific diagnosis having been made. As obesity can be such a major problem in this condition and the children need special help and management for many of their complications, we describe this particular obesity syndrome in more detail here and outline management in later chapters.

Prader–Willi syndrome

Table 5.7 lists some of the varied clinical features associated with PWS (Gunay-Aygun *et al.* 2001). The condition results from either deletion of genetic material or maternal uniparental disomy (both chromosome sections from the same parent) on the long arm of chromosome 15. It is important that the specific diagnosis is made as early as possible since growth hormone treatment is now accepted as a useful adjunct to management in this condition. Growth hormone can improve linear growth and helps weight

Table 5.7. Clinical features of Prader–Willi syndrome

Facies	Narrow forehead
	Almond-shaped eyes
	Down-turned mouth
	Triangular upper lip; 'carp-like' mouth
	Upturned retroussé nose
	High arched palate
Musculo-skeletal	Central origin muscular hypotonia
	Scoliosis
	Small hands and feet
	Flat ulnar border to hands
	Tapering fingers and toes
	Short stature
Hypothalamic abnormalities	Cryptorchidism
	Micropenis
	Small female genitalia
	Delayed or absent pubertal development
	Primary or secondary amenorrhoea
Psychodevelopmental problems	Delayed motor development
	Delayed language development
	Learning difficulties
	Cognitive difficulties
	Temper tantrums
	Controlling/manipulative behaviours
	Food seeking behaviour
	Stubbornness
Cutaneous problems	Self-inflicted wounds on arms particularly
	Intertrigo in fatfolds with secondary *Candida* infection
	Phlebitis and ulceration of oedematous legs
Nutritional state	Feeding problems in early life: failure to thrive
	Later insatiable appetite: gross obesity
Co-morbidities	Cardiorespiratory problems
	Obstructive sleep apnoea
	Type 2 diabetes melllitus
	Osteoporosis

management but is most effective when given in early life (Davies *et al.* 1998; Carrel *et al.* 2004).

Children with PWS have many problems requiring specialist supervision, usually from a multidisciplinary team (Eiholzer and Whitman 2004), but the burden of day-to-day management of weight control may fall, in the absence of alternatives, on primary and community care. In infancy these children are significantly affected by floppiness and feeding difficulties leading to failure to thrive and delayed motor milestones. As preschool children they show increasing obesity, food seeking behaviour, temper tantrums and some developmental delay. At school cognitive and learning skills are poor and they usually need a lot of educational support. In adolescence poor pubertal development, complications from gross obesity and often very difficult behaviour create major problems for clinical management. Some PWS individuals achieve skills levels that enable them to be employed but the majority of PWS adults require sheltered accommodation. Early death from cardiorespiratory or diabetic complications or from septicaemia often secondary to infected leg ulcers induced by skin picking is common (Schrander-Stumpel *et al.* 2004). Prader–Willi syndrome is not a happy condition but impressive results have been obtained by growth hormone therapy since, with strict weight control, this seems to contribute to improved behaviour and greater acquisition of useful skills (Whitman *et al.* 2002; Eiholzer *et al.* 2003).

Prader–Willi syndrome family support groups can be a useful resource to back up support from health and educational services (Prader–Willi Syndrome Association 2007). We discuss PWS further in chapters dealing with the management of obesity.

Recommendations

- We have indicated the need for children with obesity to be examined medically at the beginning of management preferably by clinicians experienced both with children and with assessing the obese.
- Whilst a normal clinic can assess most of these children using the usual range of equipment, children at the extremes of weight or age or those with physical problems will need special attention. So we suggest the following equipment for any clinic planning to manage obese and overweight children.
  (1) Scales. Anthropometric equipment for assessing obesity must be able to accommodate children of large size at any age. They should allow the subject to sit so children with physical problems can be weighed without difficulty. Beam balance weighing scales or accurate electronic scales weighing up to at least 125 kg are essential. For greater weights than this it may be necessary to use industrial scales. Scales reading up to 20 kg which weigh infants and young children who are not standing are also needed.

    Measuring weight. Children should ideally be weighed in under-clothing without shoes. If they are not prepared to undress they should be asked to remove heavy outer garments and shoes. Preferably weighing should always take place at the same time of day using the same scales and encouraging the subject to stand on the same spot on the scales. Weighing the overweight child more frequently than once a week should be discouraged. Home scales are rarely accurate enough to record day-to-day changes in weight and the slightly varying results they produce can give rise to joy one day and disappointment the next as weights are recorded as less or more than the previous occasion. Over one week, significant weight change on the scales is likely to be reflecting, with reasonable accuracy, what is happening to the body weight.

(2) Stadiometer/length measuring board. An accurate stadiometer which records standing height and a board for measuring length in children under 2 years is needed since weight must be assessed in relation to height/length.

Measuring height and length. Height measurements are made without shoes. Two people are required for accurate height measurements.

Height. The child stands looking at a fixed point ahead with feet parallel if possible, and heels, buttocks, shoulders and back of head touching the upright of the stadiometer. One person holds the feet lightly in place to stop the child rising up on to the toes. The other person tips the head usually slightly forwards by gentle upward pressure under the mastoid processes on both sides until the lower borders of the orbits and the central point of the external auditory meatus (on the side where the measurer is standing) are in the same horizontal plane (Frankfort plane). If possible get the child to breathe in as the measurement is about to be made but this can make the process too difficult for young children. The height is then read. Ideally the measurement used is the mean of at least three readings consistently within 1 mm of each other.

Length. The child is placed supine on the measuring board. One technician holds the head against the fixed head end of the board with the Frankfort plane vertical this time. The other technician holds the lower legs so that one hand gently presses the knees down towards the board and stretches the legs out straight at the same time. The foot board is brought up against the soles of the feet pressing them gently until they are at right angles to the board and the measurement is read. As with height, taking the result of several consistent readings is ideal.

(3) Waist circumference tape measure (see Chapter 2 for waist measurement). A plasticized, non-stretchable, accurate measuring tape which records in centimetres should be used to measure waist circumferences. Specially designed waist tapes can be used but are not essential. If the waist tapes are marked with 'normal' and 'overweight'

circumferences on them it must be remembered that these are (usually) values for adults not children.

(4) Centile charts for weight, height, waist circumferences for boys and girls birth to 18 years.

   Weight and height/length charts (Harlow Printing Company 2007)

   BMI charts (Harlow Printing Company 2007)

   Waist circumference centile charts (Child Growth Foundation 2007).

(5) Sphygmomanometer with a range of cuffs of different sizes.

(6) Skinfold calipers. Though as we explained in Chapter 2, we do not find skinfold measurements useful in assessing childhood obesity. Skinfold centiles for British children are very out of date (Tanner and Whitehouse 1975).

6

What complications should we look for now and later?

Obesity in childhood is not simply a matter of being too fat. In UK and many other countries conditions previously associated with adult obesity are now seen not only in obese adolescents but in quite young children (Pinhas-Hamiel *et al.* 1996). With many of these children there may be a genetic predisposition to the medical complication (for example an underlying familial hyperlipidaemia or a family history of type 2 diabetes) but the child's obesity precipitates clinical manifestations of disease decades earlier than would have been expected had there been no obesity. Not all studies are so gloomy (Srinivasan *et al.* 2003; Lawlor *et al.* 2006) but it has been suggested that a consequence of the high prevalence of obesity and its co-morbidities in childhood, if these persist, will be a fall in the mean lifespan of the current generation of children compared with that expected for their parents (Olshansky *et al.* 2005). Table 6.1 lists some of the complications which may develop or be exacerbated by obesity in childhood. In Chapter 5 we outlined some specific points in the clinical examination of obese children which included looking for clinical signs of these conditions. Here we elaborate on the conditions that may be found and their implications.

Orthopaedic problems

Non-specific aches and pains are not uncommon amongst obese children. These may be due to the weight of the child putting a strain on joints and ligaments or they may be the consequence of mild exercise in children whose lifestyle has made them unfit and thus uncomfortable with even minor activity. Occasionally muscular pains are exaggerated or fabricated in the expectation of being excused the misery of physical education (PE) and the undressing which may accompany this at school, or other activity at home. However such pains should not be glossed over as the inevitable consequences of overweight since occasionally they are symptoms of important

Table 6.1. Conditions that complicate overweight/obesity in childhood and adolescence

Orthopaedic problems	Flat feet
	Blount's disease
	Genu valgum
	Slipped upper (capital) femoral epiphysis
Skin conditions	Intertrigo
	Candida infection
	Acanthosis nigricans
	Striae
Cardiorespiratory problems	Increased prevalence of asthma
	Obstructive sleep apnoea syndrome
	Hypertension
	Pulmonary hypertension and cor pulmonale
	Pickwick syndrome
Metabolic problems	Type 2 diabetes mellitus
	Hepatosteatosis
	Hyperinsulinaemic syndrome/metabolic syndrome
	Polycystic ovary syndrome (PCOS)
Other	Pseudotumor cerebri

orthopaedic conditions. Table 6.1 includes some of the orthopaedic problems for which the overweight and obese are particularly at risk.

Flat feet

Many obese children have 'collapsed arches'. These may cause few problems but can contribute to ungainly gait and therefore teasing.

Blount's disease

This condition is not common but 60% to 80% of cases are reported as occurring in obese children (Henderson 1992). The condition results from abnormal growth in the proximal medial tibial epiphysis (Thompson and Carter 1990). The leg or, since the condition is commonly bilateral, both legs, become progressively more angulated laterally at the knee. The appearance is of bowed legs although the condition differs from rickets and some osteogenic dysplasias in that the shafts of the bones are normal in shape. The alignment of the tibia in relation to the femur gives the bowed appearance. The problem can develop at any age in childhood although onset is often divided into early (1–3 years), juvenile (4–10 years) and adolescent

(>11 years) (Dietz *et al.* 1982). Whilst Blount's disease is worth diagnosing because of the difficulties in ambulation it may cause, spontaneous cure by the age of 40 is quite common even with adolescent onset. Vigorous weight control is the most important aspect of management since, whilst surgery may be deemed appropriate, relapse after surgery is likely if the children do not lose weight.

Genu valgum

In contrast to Blount's disease we have found that many obese older children have some degree of 'knock knees' or genu valgum and may be unable to stand with their feet together as a consequence. Older children and young adolescents with very severe obesity seem the most likely to be affected. Possibly genu valgum develops as a consequence of internal rotation of the knees occurring subconsciously so as to reduce the discomfort of fat inner thighs rubbing together.

Slipped upper (capital) femoral epiphysis

Slipped upper femoral epiphysis (SUFE) is the most worrying orthopaedic problem likely to develop in overweight children. If it occurs acutely the child will have sudden severe hip pain which draws attention to the problem (Loder *et al.* 1993). If the slippage is partial, chronic less severe pain in the hip or referred pain in the ipsilateral knee can easily be attributed to non-specific aches and pains of overweight. The diagnosis of SUFE should be considered in any young adolescent with obesity, hip or knee pain and a limp. Children with hypothyroidism and hypercortisolism have increased risk of SUFE. Thyroid function tests should probably be checked in any child with SUFE. Failure to diagnose and treat SUFE early can lead to a lifelong limp and/or early osteoarthritis in the affected hip. The condition may be bilateral (Sørensen 1968; Wilcox *et al.* 1988).

Skin problems

Minor skin problems are common. These may be chafing of the skin from tight clothes rubbing fat limbs; intertrigo, sometimes exacerbated by *Candida* infection, in pendulous folds of fat around chest or abdomen; and white or pale pink striae around abdomen and upper thighs. These latter are harmless but unsightly.

In the grossly obese there may be dependent oedema with permanently swollen feet and ankles. Poor circulation to the skin of the lower limbs in association with dependent oedema may be associated with ulcers on the shins, poor healing, cellulitis or even septicaemia.

Acanthosis nigricans

This is a velvety thickening of the skin with brown to black hyperpigmentation usually in flexural areas and on pressure points. The back of the neck is a common site but areas in the axillae and on the elbows are not unusual. The condition is seen in a variety of clinical states apart from obesity including in pre-cancerous states. In childhood the condition does not usually have malign significance but can be a manifestation of hyperinsulinaemia and thus an indicator for type 2 diabetes. Not all studies show this association. It is thought that insulin binds to insulin-like growth factor receptors on the keratinocytes and fibroblasts in the dermis stimulating epidermal hyperplasia and a 'mamillated' hypertrophied epidermis overlaid by thickened stratum corneum (Richards *et al.* 1985).

Cardiorespiratory complaints

Breathlessness is commonly associated with obese individuals taking exercise. Cardiorespiratory problems range from abnormal increases in pulse and respiratory rates on minor exertion to life-threatening respiratory impairment and cardiac failure.

Lack of physical fitness and the physical effort required for minor movement by a very heavy individual explain some of the breathlessness in obesity (Eston *et al.* 1990). Obesity can create a vicious circle of high energy expenditure and effort for exercise so exercise is reduced, physical fitness declines and activity becomes even more difficult – so obesity increases. One aspect of management is to break into this cycle and increase fitness so physical activity becomes easier, fitness increases further, activity improves further – and so on.

Doppler ultrasound studies of the hearts of obese children show, as with obese adults, thickening of the left ventricular wall and the intraventricular septum in many cases (Poskitt *et al.* 1987). The significance of this is unclear but it suggests a burden on the heart from overweight and might presage future cardiac 'events'.

Asthma

Asthma is more common in overweight than normal weight children so the obese with breathlessness, especially when it occurs with exertion, should be checked for bronchospasm and lowered peak flow rate. Treating asthma could help increase affected children's abilities to exercise and thus help reduce their obesity. Reducing the obesity can help the asthma (Belamarich *et al.* 2000).

Sleep disordered breathing

Sleep disordered breathing in overweight children takes several forms. Snoring is common in all children. In sleep pharyngeal muscles relax and the airways narrow leading to the propensity for snoring, especially if there is already some obstruction to the airway from enlarged tonsils and adenoids.

Obstructive sleep apnoea syndrome

In obesity the weight of fat around the neck can cause increased pressure on the relaxed pharyngeal wall so that there is partial obstruction during respiration. Inadequate ventilation leads to – often noisy – physical effort to breathe, falls in oxygenation during sleep in association with apnoeic episodes and brief arousal with the respiratory effort. Snoring associated with obstructive apnoea affects perhaps 1% of children. It seems significantly more common amongst overweight children with prevalence in different studies ranging from <20% to >60% of overweight children. Obstructive sleep apnoea syndrome (OSAS) can be defined as

- obstructive apnoea/hypopnoea lasting >10 seconds or more than two normal respiratory cycles
- +/– age specific associated bradycardia or tachycardia
- +/– desaturation below 89% oxygenation.

Verhulst *et al.* (2007) and others have found that the prevalence of OSAS is higher in children with overweight than those classed as obese. They suggest that the energy expended fighting obstructed inspiration reduces the excess of energy intake over expenditure in these children and consequently the rate of weight increase. Removal of the tonsils reduces the efforts needed to breathe. This sounds a surprising explanation but tonsillar enlargement is very common in OSAS and for these children, tonsillectomy is first-line management for OSAS. Tonsillectomy is often documented as leading to overweight so there may be some justification for this suggestion (Verhulst *et al.* 2007). This is rather different from the usual explanation that appetite improves after the removal of large tonsils and thus energy intake is liable to become excessive.

Central sleep apnoea

In addition to OSAS, overweight/obese children are at risk of central apnoea. This can be associated with more severe desaturation and, unlike OSAS, the frequency and severity of apnoea correlate with the degree of overweight. The explanation for central sleep apnoea is far from clear. Reduced intrathoracic volume due perhaps to the weight of fat around the chest causing lower oxygen reserves, impaired central responses to hypercapnia and hypoxia, or leptin resistance are included in the many explanations.

Children with sleep disordered breathing may present with a history of snoring, restless sleep with frequent brief waking, and daytime sleepiness, irritability and inattention (Kotagal and Pianosi 2006). The extent to which sleep disturbances – whether secondary to obesity or not – may contribute to poor daytime attentiveness is uncertain but poor school progress is a potential long-term consequence of this problem (American Thoracic Society 1999; Hill *et al.* 2006). For children with OSAS and enlarged tonsils and adenoids, removal of these is an early approach to management. Urgent fat reduction should also be part of management. The following are indications for considering referral of a child for sleep and respiratory function investigations (Deane and Thomson 2006; Kotagol and Pianosi 2006):

- waking unrefreshed: morning headaches or nausea and vomiting
- undue sleepiness in classroom, falling asleep in class, on short journeys or napping at home
- habitual snoring and excessive nocturnal restlessness
- observed episodes of obstructed respiration and apnoea
- symptoms suggestive of nocturnal asthma but not responding to conventional treatment
- persistent difficulty falling asleep or staying asleep
- unexplained night time behaviours which disturb the rest of the family.

Periodic hypoxia and hypercapnia from sleep apnoea and inadequate ventilation can lead to both systemic hypertension and pulmonary artery narrowing with pulmonary hypertension. One outcome is cor pulmonale secondary to the effects of obesity.

Obesity hypoventilation syndrome (Pickwickian syndrome)

This is one of the few real emergencies in childhood obesity. Happily it is a rare occurrence in children although not uncommon amongst morbidly obese adults. Affected children are usually grossly overweight and present with history of sleep disordered breathing, polycythaemia, hypoxia and hypercapnia, signs of pulmonary hypertension and right-sided cardiac failure (Riley *et al.* 1976; Deane and Thomson 2006). On examination they may be breathless secondary to the cardiac failure but with hypoventilation. The condition may result from the great weight of fat around the chest which has to be moved with each respiration so the body makes less respiratory effort, carbon dioxide builds up and ceases to drive respiration. Build-up of carbon dioxide leads to oxygen lack rather than carbon dioxide excess driving respiration. However there are suggestions that central unresponsiveness to leptin is contributing to the hypoventilation. Whatever the cause, these children are thus at great risk when coming under medical care since administration of oxygen to relieve their respiratory symptoms may reduce the drive for respiration from oxygen lack with possible disastrous consequences. Treatment should be administered with very careful monitoring of blood gases and pH together with urgent reduction in fat mass which, at least initially, means strict dieting (Deane and Thomson 2006).

Children with PWS, partly because of their frequent gross obesity but perhaps also because of poor muscle tone and abnormal peripheral chemoreceptor responsiveness, are particularly prone to develop obesity hypoventilation syndrome. Children with Down syndrome, who are at risk of developing overweight, may have more sleep disordered breathing than average partly because of their midfacial hypoplasia and frequently marked tonsillar hypertrophy.

Hypertension

In Chapter 5 we referred to the difficulties measuring BP in obese children and in determining the significance of the pressures recorded. Definite hypertension is not uncommon in obese children particularly as they near adulthood. A diagnosis of significant hypertension should ideally only be made after recording abnormal pressures on at least two separate occasions when the child is at ease. Except in the most severe cases, vigorous efforts to reduce fat should be the first approach to management although hypertensive children should have urine checked for protein, cells and haemoglobin to screen for underlying renal problems. They should also be referred for full paediatric investigation since it could be unwise to attribute significant hypertension to obesity until other potentially treatable causes of hypertension have been excluded.

Hypertension is suggested as a complication of the hyperinsulinaemia since this can increase sympathetic activity and sodium/water retention although not all studies show the connection between insulin levels and BP. Slightly elevated BP in overweight children seems to predispose to hypertension and other complications of obesity in later life (Srinivasan *et al.* 2006).

It is interesting that two studies from Northern Ireland show how height and BMI have increased in schoolchildren over 10 years but both mean systolic and mean diastolic BP for those age groups have fallen significantly over the period (Watkins *et al.* 2004).

Hormonal and metabolic problems

Type 2 diabetes

Disconcerting reports in recent medical literature show a dramatic increase in the prevalence of type 2 diabetes (non-insulin-dependent diabetes mellitus: NIDDM) in obese children (Ehtisham and Barrett 2003; Ehtisham *et al.* 2004;

Reinehr 2005). In the UK this increase is greater amongst obese children from the ISC than amongst white children (Drake *et al.* 2002). In the USA boys of Hispanic origin seem most at risk (Shai *et al.* 2006). The condition carries a poor prognosis for ultimate health and longevity so obese children should be screened and referred for specialist advice if there is any evidence of hyperglycaemia (Viner *et al.* 2005). Ideally all obese children presenting for advice and especially adolescents and grossly obese children should have urine checked for sugar. Measurements of fasting or random blood sugar levels are advisable but these investigations will be dependent on cooperation from the child and family – and this is not always achieved. It may be necessary to wait until child and family have developed some confidence in the health professional before significant invasive investigation is possible. If there is glycosuria or a high blood sugar level, affected children should be referred to a paediatric diabetic clinic for further investigation and management. Management must include vigorous efforts to reduce BMI and fatness.

Type 2 diabetes develops as a consequence of hyperinsulinaemia and islet cell exhaustion so that the raised insulin levels are no longer able to maintain normal blood glucose levels in the presence of insulin resistance (Sabin *et al.* 2006). The role of metformin in controlling the development of insulin resistance and type 2 diabetes is currently an area of interest (Charles *et al.* 2000). However any drug treatment for these children should be only after there has been full assessment in a paediatric diabetic or endocrinology clinic.

Hyperlipidaemia

Abnormal lipid profiles are common amongst obese children. Serum cholesterol, low density lipoprotein (LDL) cholesterol and triglycerides are commonly elevated and high density lipoprotein (HDL) cholesterol levels low. Some children with abnormal lipid profiles will have familial dyslipidaemias perhaps suggested by a family history of early death or cardiovascular disease such as coronary thrombosis or stroke at a young age. Even in familial hyperlipidaemia reducing excess fat will be an important part of management. Diagnosing hyperlipidaemia can be important for advice and genetic counselling. In the absence of a suggestive family history, however, lipid profile may not be seen as an essential investigation in obese children but the knowledge that their child has risk factors resulting from obesity can give useful impetus to parents' efforts to implement healthier lifestyles.

Metabolic syndrome

The conditions of hypertension, type 2 diabetes and dyslipidaemia often overlap in obese subjects. The common factor seems to be insulin resistance to which obesity is often contributory. This clustering of insulin resistance

Table 6.2. Suggested defining features of metabolic syndrome in childhood

Children who have three or more of the following features:
- BMI >95th centile for age and gender
- Elevated fasting blood glucose
- Elevated blood glucose 2 hours after standard oral glucose tolerance test
- Systolic and/or diastolic blood pressure >90th centile for age
- HDL cholesterol <10th centile for age and gender
- Waist circumference >90th centile for age

Source: Cruz and Goran (2004).

associated problems is sometimes referred to as 'metabolic syndrome', 'syndrome X' or 'Reaven's syndrome' (Eckel *et al.* 2005; Jessup and Harrell 2005). Some clinicians question whether the clustering justifies the concept of a syndrome and there are considerable variations in the criteria used in the diagnosis (Alberti *et al.* 2005). The original description does not include central obesity.

The World Health Organization (1998) definition of metabolic syndrome in adults includes:
- type 2 diabetes or evidence of insulin resistance

plus two of the following:
- hypertension >140/90
- raised plasma triglycerides
- lowered cholesterol
- BMI >30 or raised waist : hip ratio (>0.9 in men and >0.85 in women)
- microalbuminuria; raised albumin : creatinine ratio in urine.

Other conditions such as acanthosis nigricans and polycystic ovary syndrome (PCOS) are also often linked with these features. Insulin resistance with perhaps contributing proinflammatory factors seems to underlie all the linked conditions (Eckel *et al.* 2005).

Uncertainty over the definition of metabolic syndrome, if it is a syndrome, is even greater in childhood (Cruz and Goran 2004). Clustering of metabolic problems is common although there is no strong evidence that the overall prognosis for children is worse for the combination of conditions than it would be for the conditions found individually. Making a diagnosis of possible metabolic syndrome alerts clinicians to the likelihood of a range of associated problems and the likelihood of insulin resistance and prediabetes but per se probably does not alter management.

Table 6.2 lists some criteria suggested for the definition of metabolic syndrome in childhood. Since hyperinsulinaemia seems the essential feature to all these definitions, insulin resistance syndrome of childhood may be a better term than metabolic syndrome although there is no widely accepted definition of normal insulin levels in children.

Polycystic ovary syndrome

Polycystic ovary syndrome (PCOS) is defined by irregular or absent menstruation, hyperandrogenism and polycystic ovaries on ultrasound investigation (Hopkinson *et al.* 1998; Buggs and Rosenfield 2005). Many affected girls and women are obese and there is often evidence of insulin resistance with frequent accompanying hyperlipidaemia, hypertension and even hyperglycaemia. The obesity may be contributing to the development of PCOS (which does occur in the non-obese as well) through the effects of insulin on the ovarian androgens and sex hormone binding globulin levels. Obese adolescent girls may complain of hirsutes, irregular menstruation or failure of menarche despite pubertal maturity. Acanthosis nigricans and severe acne may also cause them distress. Girls with suggestive symptomatology should be referred to a paediatric endocrinologist or adolescent gynaecological clinic.

Hepatosteatosis

Hepatomegaly seems common in obese children although clinically it is not easy to detect because of abdominal fat. Biopsy studies show excessive deposits of large fat globules in the hepatocytes (simple hepatic steatosis) and quite frequently some fibrosis (non-alcoholic steatohepatitis: NASH). Rarely the condition progresses to extensive fibrosis and ultimately cirrhosis and liver failure (Kerkar 2004; Roberts 2005).

Apart from a large liver few other clinical signs or symptoms are associated with NASH. Liver enzyme levels are usually raised. The condition is probably frequently overlooked unless there is ready access to non-invasive methods of investigation such as ultrasound and CT scanning. Reduction in the excess body fat is the main line of management and can result in total reversal if hepatic fibrosis has not developed.

Pseudotumor cerebri

Rarely obese children present with signs of raised intracranial pressure (ICP) without specific clinical reason (Dietz 1998). It has been suggested that raised ICP results from raised intrathoracic pressure secondary to raised intraabdominal pressure (Sugerman *et al.* 1999). This seems a little surprising but no better explanation has been given. Children may present with severe obesity, occipital headache, vomiting and possibly visual disturbances. They may have papilloedema and sixth nerve palsies. Unlike most children with this degree of clinical signs in association with raised ICP from other causes they are usually alert and without long tract signs. As with obesity hypoventilation syndrome, treatment is urgent weight reduction once thorough investigation has excluded other causes of raised ICP.

Recommendations

- Investigations for most overweight children should be kept to the minimum. Good history taking and full clinical assessment are adequate for children who are no more than moderately overweight and free of significant symptoms or suggestion of underlying problems. Extensive investigation can seem threatening and may deter further interest in 'doing something about the weight'.
- For the severely obese screening investigations should be indicated on clinical grounds. If there is concern that the child or adolescent is at risk of the complications of obesity (i.e. gross obesity, hypertension, family history of obesity co-morbidities for example), the following investigations may be appropriate:
  Urine:
  – cells, protein and glucose
  Blood tests:
  – haemoglobin and red blood cell count (a high haemoglobin and polycythaemia suggest chronic hypoxia)
  – fasting glucose, or if not obtainable, random blood glucose
  – fasting plasma insulin
  – serum cholesterol and lipid profile
  – liver enzymes
  Ultrasound:
  – liver size
  – cardiac size
- Other investigations such as glucose tolerance testing, computerized tomography of liver or heart or brain should be pursued through specialist paediatric units.

7

How does psychology influence management?

Research into childhood obesity has sometimes focused on searching for specific psychological traits in overweight/obese children. No consistent findings in relation to appetite and diet, physical activity or general behaviour distinguish overweight/obese children. Perhaps we should not expect findings since there is no good evidence that the obese consistently eat more or exercise less than the non-obese. However, this research was as population studies. At the individual level, particular behavioural and psychological characteristics can contribute to the development or persistence of obesity. As with everything else, each child is different.

Understanding the child in the family context

Childhood obesity is so stigmatized that it can be difficult to discuss the topic objectively – inside or outside the family or with health professionals. We have raised some of the problems parents may have acknowledging their overweight children's problems in Chapter 4. Here we look more at the attitudes and experiences of the children themselves and how these may interfere with coping with their overweight/obesity.

Challenges to psychological robustness

Children who are psychologically robust although aware of their obesity are well placed to make the lifestyle changes with which to improve their immediate or long-term health. For children who are less psychologically robust, improving their resilience when confronted with the negative perceptions of obesity amongst their peers may be the initial focus of management. Dietz (1998) has pointed out that for obese children the psychosocial consequences of being overweight/obese are worse than the risks of medical consequences.

Table 7.1. Psychological difficulties in overweight/obese children and suggestions for managing them

Problem	Possible management
Self-consciousness about obesity	Interview parents apart from children. Assess the children afterwards or at separate visits.
Low self-esteem	Identify where self-esteem can be rebuilt (academic achievement, social competences, anything the child recognizes as something worthwhile which they can do). Strengthening one competency can spread benefit to other competencies.
Low self-confidence	Identify tasks that are achievable but just outside the children's comfort zones. If tasks are not completed, the confidence building process is likely to be set back but can be rejoined at an earlier phase. If tasks are achieved, set slightly more adventurous ones each time so children develop growing sense of achievement.
Teasing/bullying	Notify the school. Work to build up self-confidence and self-esteem to counter bullying tactics. Make clear strong disapproval of any victimization of others by the obese child.
Learning difficulties	Educational psychology assessment and school support with learning needed.
Unhappiness, grief	If there is cause for grief – bereavement, family break-up – this may pass with time but parents need to make sure grief is recognized and tackled sensitively. If there is teasing or bullying causing unhappiness, tackle this. If there are educational difficulties, discuss with the school. Where there is persistent inexplicable unhappiness consider the possibility of depressive illness.
Suggestion of child abuse	Occasionally obesity is a manifestation of child (sexual) abuse. If there is any suggestion of this, alert the Child Protection Services.
Eating disorder	Seek child or adolescent psychiatric help.
Depression	Seek child or adolescent psychiatric help.

Table 7.1 lists some of the psycho-emotional strains on obese children's coping strategies. These may not only prevent successful weight control but can actually contribute to furtherance of excessive weight gain. Although we outline suggested management approaches, remedial strategies need discussion and negotiation with each child and family on an individual basis so as to determine the most appropriate way forward for that child and that family.

Teasing and bullying

Obesity is like many medical conditions in that affected children are seen by their peers as different and may be subject to teasing, bullying or ostracization. The nature of obesity makes affected children all too obvious prey for name calling, excessive teasing and verbal and physical bullying. Even so, not all children who are overweight suffer bullying or teasing or isolation. Some, particularly young obese boys, may benefit from their obesity and overall large size by being good at sport and formidable opponents in physical encounters. It might be expected, with the prevalence of overweight/obesity in the population so high, that the public image of obesity would have improved yet the negative images surrounding obesity seem to remain endemic in our society (Swallen *et al.* 2005). Children as young as 3 or 4 years old pick up disparaging remarks about overweight from older children and adults. Whilst there is little evidence that perceptions of the obese have changed in recent years, there is some evidence that the level of BMI at which obesity is recognized as such by the general public has increased. The overweight may now escape victimization but the obese remain vulnerable.

Schools in UK have policies for zero tolerance of bullying and can be good at taking action when bullying incidents come to light but it is difficult for them to enforce these policies on all occasions particularly once children are outside the school gates. The finding that baiting the obese is commonly peer group wide rather than just caused by a few bullying individuals suggests that programmes teaching peer acceptance and the promotion of diversity, including weight diversity, need to be strengthened across whole schools. Trying to pinpoint individual perpetrators may be ineffective (Hayden-Wade *et al.* 2005).

Parents are often reluctant to inform schools about bullying because they are afraid that bringing the problem into the open may make the situation worse for their children. They may be labelled as 'fussy' by teachers. Yet schools cannot be expected to act if they do not know what is happening.

Some children seem more resilient than others to teasing and bullying from their peers. Susceptibility to victimization seems partly related to the severity of the overweight/obesity. One Canadian study showed that victimization, both verbal and physical, increased with increasing levels of BMI at all ages studied (11–16 years) except amongst teenage boys where physical victimization of the overweight was not increased compared to that of the normal weight. This particular finding might be explained by the 'overweight' group of male adolescents including some very muscular, mature but not obese, boys with whom other boys might feel it foolish to engage. Appearance related teasing can induce great anxiety about weight, exacerbate body dissatisfaction, loneliness and isolation from social activities and lead to a preference for lone sedentary 'activity' (Hayden-Wade *et al.* 2005).

None of these associations is likely to benefit obese children struggling to control their weight. Their response to their own victimization may be to take on the role of bully or to play truant. The Canadian study cited above found both 15–16-year-old obese boys and obese girls were more likely than normal weight children of that age to be the perpetrators of victimization. Similar findings were apparent in the Avon Longitudinal Study of Parents and Children (ALSPAC) where obese boys of primary school age were 1.66 times more likely than any other group to be overt bullies, presumably due to their physical dominance. However in this age group other obese boys seem just as likely to be victims as girls (Griffiths *et al.* 2006). Inappropriate behaviours can develop as a result of the negative social effects of the victimization and rejection by peers experienced by some obese children (Janssen *et al.* 2006). Further increases in the severity of obesity seem almost inevitable when children become lonely and isolated.

Developing coping skills and resilience against teasing and bullying requires building up children's self-esteem, self-confidence and sence of self-worth. Below are suggestions for ways in which parents of obese children might help their children cope with bullying.

- Avoid all pointed remarks, teasing, joking about the child's weight from siblings and the rest of the family. Encourage positive tolerance of diversity within the family.
- Talk constructively with the child so overweight is not a hidden misery.
- Improve self-esteem by praising the child for looking smart, behaving well, showing good social relations with others etc.
- Ensure the child is appropriately clean and neat and that clothes fit so there is no justification for jibes about appearance.
- Champion the child:
     Inform the school of bullying incidents
     Consider discussing their children's behaviour with the parents of bullies.
- Help the child find resilient, supportive and loyal friends
- Build up skills by encouraging the child to take part in physical activity at home or in nearby open spaces with family or trusted friends.
- Reduce opportunities for self-pity by discouraging the child from opting out of peer group activities.
- Make it clear that any bullying behaviour by the child is totally unacceptable however much the child may have been the recipient of such behaviour.
- Take action to control weight which should improve self-esteem and remove a cause for teasing.

Self-esteem, self-worth

Self-esteem is gained from feelings of competence in a range of domains (such as physical appearance, athletic ability, social competence, intellectual

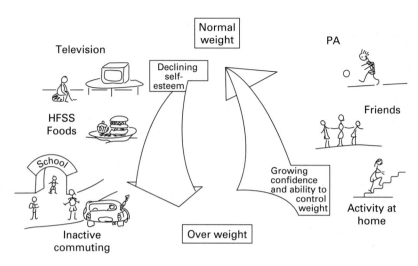

Figure 7.1 Impact of various activities on weight, self-esteem and ability to control weight. HFSS: high fat, high sugar, high salt.

ability, behavioural conduct and desirability to a partner etc.). At around 8 years of age, children can distinguish between different domains and learn to judge their competences in them (Harter 1993). Domains where children feel less competent may be discounted to preserve self-esteem. However the one domain which is rarely discounted is physical appearance and this contributes strongly to self-esteem at all ages and for both sexes. Self-worth is built up over time by exposing different competences and receiving feed back about them and relating these to societal/cultural norms (Figure 7.1). For example, children who are not good at sports can discount that domain. Their lack of prowess does not alter their self-worth. Finding skills at which the obese can excel is important in helping them value themselves more highly and give them the self-confidence to take positive action to control weight.

Not all obese children have low self-esteem (Franklin *et al.* 2006). Indeed some research data suggest that low self-esteem is no more a problem for the obese than for the non-obese. French *et al.* (1995) reviewed whether:

- low self-esteem is a constant characteristic of childhood overweight?
- any association between self-esteem and obesity is specific to physical appearance or impacts globally on self-esteem?
- high self-esteem protects against developing obesity?
- changes in self-esteem predict weight loss in treatment programmes?

Nineteen cross-sectional studies (children aged 7–12 years) showed either no significant difference or slightly lowered self-esteem amongst overweight children. No study reported a positive effect of obesity on self-esteem. Results did not seem affected by the age or sex of the children and self-esteem scores for both overweight and normal weight children all fell within the normal range. Where assessments of self-esteem were included in treatment programmes, self-esteem seemed to increase as weight was lost.

In adolescence, inverse relationships between overweight, self-esteem and body esteem seem more consistent. Higher self-esteem was associated with better weight loss but increasing adolescents' self-esteem did not necessarily produce greater weight losses. There was some evidence for high self-esteem protecting against the development of obesity in adolescence (French *et al.* 1995).

Viner *et al.* (2006) have shown that the relationship between self-esteem and obesity varies with ethnicity amongst 11–14-year-old UK children. Low self-esteem was not associated with overweight in girls but there was an association with obese boys. Within ethnic subgroups, self-esteem was significantly lower in overweight white British boys and obese boys and girls of Bangladeshi origin, but significantly higher in obese girls of Afro-Caribbean origin. In another community sample of adolescents, Wardle and Cooke (2005) found that whilst body dissatisfaction was common, few overweight or obese suffered low self-esteem and even fewer had depressive symptoms. They found three factors in obese children associated with negative effects on well-being: being female, white and adolescent. These studies show how complicated are the interactions of self-esteem and high BMI. Despite the social stigma of being overweight and high levels of body dissatisfaction, most obese adolescents cope remarkably well. Wardle and Cooke (2005) suggest that rather than concentrating on looking for childhood depression in the obese, it may be more profitable to 'identify the best means by which stigmatisation, discrimination, teasing and bullying can be reduced'. Health care practitioners have the capacity to contribute to and support such a programme.

School failure

Some overweight children are failing at school and may be victimized for this so they withdraw from their peers, exercise less and snack alone for comfort. For many of these children, the stress of trying to cope with school work precipitates the overweight rather than the other way round, although both sequences do occur. It is important to recognize those children for whom educational assessment and appropriate help with school work may aid weight control by improving self-efficacy and social development.

Unhappiness, isolation and low self-esteem

For many overweight children the emotional health related quality of life seems much the same as for non-overweight children although poor physical quality of life is a common finding amongst those overweight (Swallen *et al.* 2005; Pinhas-Hamiel *et al.* 2006). Sometimes the concept of reduced emotional quality of life is more a perception of the parents than the experience of the overweight children (Hughes *et al.* 2007). However, unhappiness, failure to integrate well within peer groups, loneliness and a feeling of low self-worth do contribute to the development of, or result from, obesity in some children. The unhappiness may have very specific and obvious cause. Actual bereavement or apparent parental desertion in a family break-up underlie the development of obesity in some. Children's distress may be overlooked in the presence of adult distress such as may accompany the death of a grandparent. In circumstances of family break-up, physical disturbances such as moving house may accompany parental emotional disturbance. Children's eating can become disturbed with little notice from parent or carers when overweight begins to develop. Parent/carer guilt or a new step-parent wanting to develop positive relationships can lead to overindulgence and consequent obesity for these children. The possibility of childhood depression should be considered when there is unhappiness persisting over months without reasonable cause.

Overindulgence or 'spoiling'

Some parental practices allow children to eat more or less what they like when they like. Overindulgence may not be simply over food. Parents may overindulge children by doing things for them when the children could easily do these things for themselves and expend energy in the process. In these ways children may develop lifestyles of being 'waited on' by parents so they have little PA, excessive television viewing, uncontrolled snacking and the presumption that what they want, they get. This too easily contributes to obesity. For other parents establishing and maintaining 'no' boundaries are difficult with adverse consequences for children's weights. Sometimes giving children opportunities to do things for themselves is a matter of finding time for the slow and initially only partly successful action by the children. In the long term, allowing time for children to develop the ability to look after themselves and to join in family activities is time well spent.

In many of these situations helping parents and children recognize how changed intra-family dynamics could create more effective management of their children's overweight requires considerable tact. The quality of the relationships between the HCPs and obese children or adolescents and their parents is critical to managing the weight problem. Health professionals often share the negative attitudes of the rest of society and may not appreciate the complexity of having an overweight child in the family. Unhelpful attitudes will come across in non-verbal communication. Findings from an interview-based study with parents of overweight children showed a range of responses from HCPs. General practitioners and other medically qualified personnel could be sympathetic, offering tests, referral and general advice but some blamed mothers, or dismissed self-help attempts to diet or to increase physical activity, or labelled mothers as 'making a fuss'. Some just showed lack of interest. Health visitors usually offered plenty of practical advice. Paediatric dietitians were child-centred and very supportive but experiences with community dieticians were less constructive (Edmunds 2005). These findings may or may not reflect others' experiences but they demonstrate the importance of the quality of interaction. They also highlight that parents may have had previous negative experiences when engaging with HCPs and effort may be required to restore confidence in the help offered.

Obesity often runs in families. In the UK the association between the prevalence of obesity and low SES seems to vary with the study (Kinra *et al.* 2000; Viner and Cole 2005). However the families of overweight/obese children will include some who are unskilled and/or socially disadvantaged. Interventions must relate to what families are likely to be able to achieve in their homes and communities and with their finances. For the parents, their own parenting, the demands of their work, their obesogenic lifestyles and perhaps low levels of education may all be factors which complicate their aspirations to improve their children's weight and lives. Gently introduced small changes in family lifestyles may be all that is possible. Yet, without some lifestyle changes involving the family, nothing is likely to be achieved. Sympathetic support may improve well-being, in itself a good thing, but may have no effect on weight.

Studies of pre-adolescent children suggest that working with the parents is the most effective way of managing childhood overweight. This does not mean disregarding the children and their problems and perceptions of obesity but rather recognizing that effective change for these children is through parental action and provision of the environment in which the child's lifestyle can change. Without this nothing is likely to be achieved. With age and increasing maturity, children and adolescents need to learn to accept responsibility for their own weight management but to recognize the help and support parents and other significant adults can give.

For each obese child and family, the advice will be different and the markers of progress will be individual. Advice may even be the wrong description of the help needed. Health care professionals should be guiding these families to find their own solutions to issues raised in discussion. It is this which requires delicacy, understanding and tact. Our recommendations may be fine in theory but if they are not implementable within the family, they will not be successful.

Improving psychological well-being is a necessary adjunct to any successful weight management strategy, is unlikely to do any harm, and may be protective against unsafe weight management practices in the child/adolescent (O'Dea 2005). The serious eating disorders are mostly associated with underlying psychotic personalities and need recognizing and referring for psychiatric management. Affected children do not necessarily have a history of overweight/obesity although that may be their concept of their nutritional state.

Psychoses

It is not clear how much overweight and obesity in childhood contribute to, or result from, psychological disorders. Significant psychopathology is less common than early work on obesity may have suggested. Vila *et al.* (2004) found psychological disturbance – usually anxiety disorders – quite commonly amongst a group of obese children and adolescents. The severity of the illness did not relate to the degree of overweight but was usually worst in the children of parents who themselves had psychological disturbances.

Eating disorders

Concern that treating obesity may precipitate eating disorders is frequently the reason given by parents, particularly mothers, for taking no action to control their children's, especially their daughters', weights. The connections between dieting and eating disorders, whilst well established in the public mind, are scientifically unclear. One study (Schleimer 1983) found no relationship, whereas two later studies (Killen *et al.* 1994; Patton *et al.* 1999) found associations between obesity in adolescent girls and the development of bulimia nervosa. Anorexia and bulimia nervosa are both characterized by exaggerated fear of gaining weight and perceiving the body to be fatter than it is – distorted body image (Nicholls and Viner 2005). Many children and adults, even though normal weight, have some body dissatisfaction and admit to longing for a slimmer (usually) figure than they have. Distorted body image is different. These sufferers perceive themselves as grossly different from what their weight and fatness indicate and the thought obsesses them.

Early concepts of anorexia nervosa were a manifestation of excessive slimming in girls who began slimming because they were obese and were overenthusiastic dieters. This overlooked the distorted body image in this condition and the need to control some aspect of their lives. Anorexics have a dread of fatness which intrudes into their whole lifestyle and is rarely related to any history of significant past overweight. Their ability to lose weight and to maintain low weight whilst pretending real enthusiasm for food and meals, together with their vigorous physical activity, contrast dramatically with the harsh reality for virtually all obese/overweight children and adolescents, namely that they have the greatest difficulty controlling their weight and, often, increasing their activity. The risk of a child developing anorexia because of sensible recommendations to control what is already excessive weight and fatness is low. A potential risk remains that their psychologically vulnerable friends may pick up ideas about dieting, decide they want to make themselves thinner and themselves progress to anorexia. For this reason those working with overweight/obese children should avoid emphasis on 'dieting' and make sure changes in eating habits are part of a range of lifestyle changes. Any change instituted should not put normal weight children at risk.

There does seem some risk of developing bulimic symptoms amongst overweight/obese children particularly adolescent girls. A focus on dieting or dietary restraint may promote a greater likelihood of bulimia in psychologically susceptible individuals/families. Bingeing on food is common in children who are perhaps dieting of their own accord and may avoid eating certain foods or meals but then make up for any physiological energy deficit by uncontrolled eating of other foods. In bulimia the bingeing is dramatic and takes place over a short space of time in adolescents or children who show obsessive interest in trying to control their intakes. The bingeing is then counteracted by self-induced vomiting, and purging if the children have the means. This combination of highly abnormal behaviours should raise concern and suggest the need for psychiatric referral.

Depression

Depression is sometimes regarded as a cause or consequence of obesity. Nutrition and depression are linked in that adult depressives who have lost weight may reduce their risk of relapse by maintaining higher body weights. Adult obesity can by contrast increase the risk of depression perhaps through the negative thoughts that go with personal isolation and the frequent failures many have experienced in attempting to lose weight. Depression does not seem to have a significant association with pre-adolescent obesity but there may be some links between depressive symptomatology and obesity in adolescence. These may be because there are factors associated with both conditions, namely declining levels of physical activity, increasing social isolation and increasing socioeconomic inequality (Goodman and Whitaker 2002). The treatment of depression should have positive effects on the management of obesity so it seems wise to consider the presence of significant psychopathology of this type underlying or developing with the obesity. If there does seem reason to consider the diagnosis of depression, child or adolescent psychiatric assessment should be sought.

Behavioural management in Prader-Willi syndrome

The strain of managing children with PWS is such that these families usually need a lot of social and psychological support and help in the form of family therapy (Forster and Gourash 2005). Children with PWS have many behavioural characteristics which make their management difficult whether or not they have need of weight control. Significant obesity as part of PWS is so common that dietary and activity controls should be part of all management programmes for these children. Overall supervision should be by professionals, often working as a multidisciplinary team, experienced with the syndrome (Eiholzer and Whitman 2004). Day-to-day management is still likely to fall on those working with the children in the community. We make a few suggestions for management here.

The behavioural difficulties of PWS children can be grouped as:
- food related behaviours
- oppositional defiance
- anxiety/insecurity
- cognitive rigidity/inflexibility
- skin picking.

The food related behaviours include:
- overeating
- unrestrained and inappropriate eating (e.g. raw, waste or pet food)
- night time foraging
- manipulative and aggressive behaviour in order to get food
- theft and dishonesty in order to obtain food (going next door and saying no one gave them breakfast)
- invasive action such as breaking locks on cupboards and refrigerators in order to obtain food.

Confronted with these problems it is easy to see why obesity prevention, difficult though it is, should be easier in the long term than trying to control obesity once it has developed. Those who have managed to control the weight of PWS children in their care often comment that overall behaviour and achievement are better in these children. In this respect treatment with growth hormone is also helpful (see Chapter 5). The overall management of PWS children can be helped by providing a daily programme of planned and supervised physical activity and occupation. A 'food security' discipline for these children is one approach to management of the eating problems (Forster and Gourash 2005). The concept is that the anxiety about obtaining food pervades these children's lives. If they are presented with a situation where the appearance of food is predictable both in time and quality and that no amount of manipulative behaviour can affect this situation, then a major reason for anxiety is eliminated. The principles of food security for PWS are that there shall be:

- no doubt when meals will occur and what foods will be served
- no hope of getting anything different from what is planned
- no disappointment related to false expectations.

This regime puts enormous strains on families and carers but is an improvement on the chaotic home life and constant verbal and even physical confrontations which are the reality for many PWS children's families. In practice a food security regime involves:

- avoiding situations where children will be unnecessarily confronted by food
- keeping food locked up
- preventing opportunities for the children to buy food (such as pocket money controls)
- supervising children not only in the home but in the community
- displaying a family menu prepared beforehand so children know what they will be eating
- avoiding unplanned eating events
- providing consistent meals and portion sizes.

For these children the need to provide food to satisfy their often voracious appetites but also to keep energy intakes in control leads to recommendations for a balance of nutrients rather different from that recommended for normal children. The bulk of meals and snacks should be as vegetables and fruits in at least six servings per day. Bread, pasta, cereals and potatoes are served less frequently and in modest amounts. At least half the meal plate should be vegetables (or fruit) with no more than a quarter plate for staple, a quarter for meat/fish, etc (Ekaitis 2007). This PWS 'food pyramid' can be followed beneficially by all obese children.

Recommendations

- Assessment of overweight/obese children needs to consider the psycho-social issues that may impact on these children's well-being. The problems may be clear cut and manageable. Action may be needed to put a stop to bullying at school. Advice may be needed over poor school progress. For the other emotional problems positive reinforcement of the children's skills and abilities is often what is necessary. If children can implement some weight control, this can improve self-confidence, sense of self-worth and resilience in the face of teasing.

- Discussions with overweight/obese children and their families should always use language which is as supportive as possible for children who may have low self-esteem or who may be very sensitive about their size.
- Group activities, group programmes and summer camps for those willing and able to attend can help promote self-esteem and sense of self-worth and can enhance physical skills. Amongst their overweight peers, children may succeed where they have previously failed and may improve skills untroubled by name calling and physical victimization. They return home with improved physical prowess, enhanced self-esteem and greater self-confidence with which to face adverse comments from their schoolmates.
- When behaviour or symptoms suggest the possibility of psychosis, referral for child or adolescent psychiatric help is essential – as would be the case for the non-obese child.
- All those working with the obese have a role in promoting policies of no discrimination on grounds of appearance. Avoiding unjustified comments against the obese has not always been perceived as relevant or put into practice with these policies.
- The increase in both obesity and depression in adults with reduced physical activity in modern society suggests there is work to be done in increasing the opportunities for physical activity – for children in safe places after school hours and in reducing the social isolation of both overweight adults and children within our societies.

8

Management: what do we mean by lifestyle changes?

In simple terms control of overweight and obesity requires a sustained period of energy expenditure exceeding energy intake. Overweight individuals' dietary intakes and activity levels have to change. However, overweight and obesity arise because energy balance has been influenced by the environment – family and community – in which the obese live. Without changes in these environments, weight control is unlikely to be sustained for long. Thus, almost inevitably, successful weight control involves behavioural changes for the family as well as for the overweight child. Further, since evidence suggests that 'healthier' lifestyles can reduce morbidity risks for the overweight/obese even without significant change in weight status, the prime aim of management should be to develop healthier behaviours. Appropriate weight controlling strategies can then be incorporated into these (Avenell *et al.* 2006).

If we consider programmes which aim to control overweight and obesity in children, some are impressively successful. Others are not. Overall, obesity management programmes have a reputation for disappointing outcomes. The fault may not always lie in the programme itself but in the way in which it is implemented (or not implemented).

Table 8.1 suggests some reasons why well-planned schemes may appear to have little effect on childhood overweight. There is no consensus on how or where overweight and obesity in childhood (or even in adult life) should be managed (Chapter 3). Factors such as the severity of the overweight, the enthusiasm, or not, of the children to focus on weight control and the social circumstances of children and their families are only some of the elements which influence the success or otherwise of attempted weight management. Some aspects of weight management can be influenced by community, media and even governmental action so as to promote positive societal change. However most of these changes apply as much to prevention as to management of overweight/obesity and are discussed in Chapter 13. The lifestyle changes we discuss here are largely those involving intra-family behaviour and aspirations.

Table 8.1. Why do treatment programmes for childhood overweight and obesity fail?

Ad hoc programmes which:
- fail to investigate the target population to find out what help is needed and how to deliver it
- lack evaluation of programme including feedback from participants

Unreasonable expectations for:
- what can be achieved
- the time period of achievement

Limited targets for interventions:
- only energy intakes targeted
- only energy expenditure targeted
- focus on overall energy balance without attention to family dynamics and lifestyle
- failure to involve whole family and/or school in process of weight control
- weight loss/reduction in BMI seen as the goal rather than acquisition of a healthier lifestyle

Advice poorly tailored to individuals and their families:
- inappropriate advice for age and independence of children
- inappropriate advice for particular family socioeconomic circumstances. e.g. both parents working; no garden; city high rise apartment

Advisors fail to recognize the difficulties some families have (SES; family set-up; control over children)

Failure of some subjects to acknowledge they have a problem which needs treatment so they disregard all advice

How much should families be involved in weight control?

Family commitment to help overweight children is vital. How families are involved depends on the children's ages and independence but without families leading behavioural change weight change in the children is unlikely to be sustainable (Edmunds *et al.* 2001; Golan and Crow 2004; McGarvey *et al.* 2004; Edwards *et al.* 2006). Even with older children and adolescents, parents have an important supporting role. They are also likely to prepare most meals and to control the family shopping basket. Siblings and other relatives can affect the self-confidence and self-esteem of the overweight by jeering, teasing or simply tempting them with inappropriate food. Family policy should include zero tolerance for this sort of sibling strife. Where practical the whole family should adapt a weight controlling lifestyle and make at least some contributory dietary changes since the prevalence of overweight in families suggests that all may benefit from changed lifestyles. Negotiations may be required with grandparents and other members of the extended family over 'treats' for the children.

Table 8.2. Lifestyle changes parents could promote to help overweight/obese children

Encourage activities, mental, physical and social, to discourage thoughts of food
Encourage socialization within families: do things with families and/or friends
Encourage children to join in simple domestic activity:
• bedmaking, tidying bedroom
• washing up/loading and unloading dishwasher
• simple cookery
• gardening activities
• fetching and carrying for others
• simple errands: walking the dog
Develop hobbies: even sedentary hobbies may divert children's thoughts from snacking
Encourage activity: use stairs, walk, cycle, use public transport not family car
Encourage personal responsibility and appropriate independence but guide children about controlling the snacking which independence makes more available
Encourage 'healthy' use of television (see Table 8.4)
Develop a bedtime policy
Lower the central heating

Suggesting non-edible items or activities as alternatives to edible treats may be more acceptable and constructive than denying all treats. All recommendations for the management of overweight and obesity should be compatible with sustainable, healthy but also happy, lifestyles for normal weight siblings as well as overweight children.

What behavioural changes should take place?

Table 8.2 suggests possible lifestyle changes which could contribute to developing healthier lifestyles. Parents are important role models. More communal activities as a family can lead to the overweight having more 'outgoing' lives with less time spent focusing on food (assuming that communal family activities do not include visits to the local burger bar!). In some families the need to aspire to better interpersonal communication within the home and to provide more stimulus and activity for their children is not recognized or accepted. Current sociological studies suggest that communication between parents and children through, for example, speech and play is very important for optimal child development (Dietz 2001). Television is no substitute for this nor for imaginative play.

Sleep

Some studies suggest that children who sleep less are at above average risk of obesity (Chaput *et al.* 2006; Taheri 2006). This is an interesting finding which could have some significance for the present epidemic rise in childhood over-weight and obesity (Astrup 2006). There is little precise documentation but it is an impression that many children have less formalized 'bedtimes' than in the past. There are a number of possible reasons for this including the almost uni-versal presence of television and the fact that many children watch television, DVDs or videos, perhaps in their bedrooms, until late at night. A more relaxed approach to child rearing with less structured parenting – in this instance over specified bedtimes – may be another explanation. Parents who are working all day may also want to spend more time with their children in the evenings than in the past when mothers had often been at home with the children around them for most of the day and might perhaps have looked forward to child-free evenings.

The physiological effects of sleep on weight control are independent of the obvious situation that if children are asleep they are not eating although both this and reduced activity during the day due to increased tiredness could contribute to the effect (Taheri 2006). Short sleep duration leads to lower levels of circulating leptin and higher levels of ghrelin. Leptin levels reflect the quantity of adipose tissue in the body and regulate energy balance within the body by suppressing appetite and stimulating energy expenditure. Ghrelin is formed in the gastric mucosa and is elevated during hunger but falls on eating (Meier and Gressner 2004). It has almost the opposite effect on appetite to leptin thus adding to the effects of short sleep duration on appetite (Taheri 2006).

There are no specific recommendations for children's bedtimes. Parents who are trying to control their children's weights should consider taking a firmer line about bedtime and 'lights out'. Maybe bedtime cannot be made earlier than at present but perhaps it should be some time before it is made any later. And 'bedtime' should mean bedtime and not time spent playing with gizmos in the bedroom.

One aspect of child obesity prevalence which is difficult to explain is the varied distribution of obesity across Europe. The UK has a prevalence which is high compared with the Scandinavian countries but below that for much of Southern Europe (Lobstein and Frelut 2003). It is an impression that children in Southern Europe are often awake very late, eating with their parents at 10 or 11 in the evening. Is obesity prevalent in these countries because many children have insufficient sleep? We do not know.

Television

Studies in several countries, including the USA, the UK, Mexico, Thailand, New Zealand and Australia, have shown that the prevalence of obesity in a study group correlates with the time the study children spend watching television (Robinson *et al.* 1993; Gortmaker *et al.* 1996; Hernandez *et al.* 1999; Wake *et al.* 2003; Hancox and Poulton 2006). The correlations between hours spent watching television and overweight may be more significant for girls than for boys. In New Zealand, Hancox *et al.* (2004) estimated that time spent watching television was a more significant predictor of BMI than diet or physical activity. For young adults, watching television for more than 2 hours a day contributed to greater overweight, higher serum cholesterol, more smoking and reduced fitness (Hancox and Poulton 2006). The epidemic rise in childhood obesity in UK has roughly paralleled rises in the number of hours television programmes are available, the number of channels available and the opportunities to watch DVDs and videos as well as television. To this we must now add the opportunities to view programmes on a wide range of equipments as well as the family television. Are all these rises in viewing opportunities coincidental or is television a very significant factor in the development of an overweight population in the UK?

Initial studies of adolescent American boys showed greater levels of obesity amongst those watching most television per week (Dietz and Gortmaker 1985). These authors estimated that the prevalence of obesity amongst 12–17-year-old boys increased by 2% for every additional hour of television viewed per day. Time spent watching television could be displacing more active pastimes and encouraging snacking. High levels of television viewing seem to be associated with greater consumption of high fat, high sugar, high salt (HFSS) foods in meals and snacks and less fruit and vegetables (Coon *et al.* 2001; Coon and Tucker 2002). Any weight gain may relate more to the snacks consumed than to low energy expenditure whilst viewing. Advertising on television may also influence dietary habits, and meal skipping or rushing meals seems more common in adolescents who watch more television (van den Buick and Eggermont 2006). Further, television encourages sedentariness. The effect of television viewing on resting energy expenditure probably varies with individuals in that some may be much more 'at rest' and sedentary than others (Klesges *et al.* 1993; Cooper *et al.* 2006). Cochrane Reviews of prevention and treatment of overweight/obesity in children suggest that reducing sedentary behaviour such as watching television can help weight management (Summerbell *et al.* 2003, 2005).

Table 8.3 lists some reasons why television viewing may contribute to overweight/obesity. Being sedentary and being physically active seem to have different motivations. Although children are often relatively active or relatively sedentary, some physically very active children also watch a lot of television (Biddle *et al.* 2004; Hesketh *et al.* 2006). Children with a high viewing rate are not necessarily unfit (Grund *et al.* 2001). So the effects of television viewing on weight are complex, acting through time spent with low energy expenditure whilst viewing, the consumption of high energy snacks

Table 8.3. Why might television contribute to overweight/obesity?

The viewer is usually sedentary

Time spent watching takes away from time that could be spent in physical activity

Eating in front of the television as an individual:

- may mean that the volumes consumed are largely unnoticed
- satisfaction from food may be less because it is consumed largely unnoticed
- food available whilst viewing more likely to involve consumption of high energy snacks and sweetened drinks

Eating in front of the television as a family:

- may reduce inter-family socializing and lead to less satisfaction from the meal
- may encourage use of (possibly energy dense) prepared meals which can be microwaved in between programmes or presentations of snacks, rather than possibly more satisfying home-cooked meals

Food advertising on television may influence consumption adversely

Television may enhance fear of the world outside the home thus discouraging outdoor physical exercise and growing independence in the children

---

whilst watching and the impact of the food advertising associated with commercial channels. We discuss food advertising in Chapter 13 on the prevention of obesity.

Exerting some control on the time children spend watching television seems likely to help weight control. Probably the least confrontational way of doing this if children already have established viewing habits, is to introduce other activities as a family so overweight children have less time – and perhaps ultimately less interest – in finding entertainment from television. In other words, encourage play (Dietz 2001). This may not be practical for all busy families. Table 8.4 suggests some principles for television use which may help in weight control. Food eaten whilst viewing may be less noticed and therefore either less satisfying or more easily consumed in excess than home-prepared meals served at table in the company of the family. Eating and drinking whilst viewing need to be restricted. The whole family needs to participate in 'healthy' viewing (at least until the children have gone to bed) since it is unreasonable to expect overweight children to behave very differently from their siblings 'because of their weight'.

What is the impact of computer and computer games on weight control?

Computers may involve slightly greater energy expenditure than that spent watching television particularly when digital games are being played (Kautianinen *et al.* 2005). However playing computer games takes time when this could be spent in more active pursuits. Manipulating a computer uses

Table 8.4. Suggestions for healthy management of television viewing in childhood

Encourage children to watch specific programmes rather than turn on television for entertainment without a specific programme in mind

Restrict maximum number of hours children watch per day and per week

No television in bedroom

No eating whilst watching: drinks confined to water, unsweetened dilute fruit squash or tea or coffee with no sugar

Television off during mealtimes

Parents find time and interest to watch television with children and discuss programmes, especially advertisements and significance of advertisements. Where practical, try to turn interest of programmes into active play

Use family time to play games and develop hobbies rather than spend it watching television

Make sure homework is completed before children watch television so bedtimes are not delayed after television because homework still has to be done

Avoid using television or video as a babysitter to keep young children quiet and 'out of mischief'

the hands which may prevent the excess of snacking that can occur whilst watching television. At the same time computer users do not suffer the barrage of food advertising which dominates commercial breaks on television. Nevertheless, time spent in front of the computer could be time spent in PA. Whether we shall see greater energy expenditure at computers or even greater physical exercise in sport as a result of the new game playing computer programs such as Wii (Nintendo: Tokyo, Japan) has yet to be seen. These computer games present opportunities to participate in a variety of 'virtual' sports (such as golf, fishing, boxing). The handset of the equipment demands fairly realistic movements and considerable physical effort in order to swing the 'virtual' golf club or to box with the 'virtual' gloved fist. Perhaps the effort involved will increase the energy expended in computer games. Ideally the games will be so realistic that the players will go on to take up the real sport.

Environmental temperature

Today the majority of homes in the UK have some form of central heating as do most public buildings. This has not always been so. Energy expended keeping warm may form only a small proportion of total energy expenditure most of the year. However, it may have contributed significantly towards energy expenditure in the past. It could help weight control if families lower the thermostats at home, cut down the hours of central heating and adopt warmer clothing instead. Ensuring children are active around the home will help keep them warm even when the house is a little cool. We acclimatize to environmental temperatures but by energy expenditure. Even if lowering the thermostat has no noticeable effect on the overweight child it may benefit fuel bills and is an appropriate action when global warming is creating so much public concern.

Particular groups

The young preschool child

Preschool children are notorious for their determination, displays of negative behaviour and ability to use manipulative behaviour with their parents. These skills are difficult to manage for all families with young children. Trying to implement diet and activity change on top of the problems caused by usual toddler behaviour can seem a nightmare to already fraught and frustrated parents. Yet this age, when children are still almost entirely dependent on their parents/carers for food and opportunities for vigorous exercise would seem an ideal age for successful implementation of healthy lifestyles. Suggestions to families of overweight young children for reducing management difficulties are:

- Discuss the rationale for change with the children in positive ways that they may be able to understand.
- Recognize that in this age group a decision or choice has none of the meaning that it has for older children. Choice can be confusing and is not perceived as being a commitment to something or some activity. Significant changes may be achieved more readily if not presented as choices.
- Make it clear to the child that a parental 'No' means 'No' and not 'I'll give in if you go on asking long enough,' i.e. establish and maintain 'No' boundaries.
- Avoid presenting change when children are tired and likely to be less cooperative.
- Avoid confronting children with change when they are very hungry and again less likely to cooperate.
- Participate in change yourself – or at least when the children are watching. (Parents who do not eat vegetables cannot expect their children to eat vegetables.)
- Do not be put off. Children may refuse new foods many times before accepting the foods. They may express disgust at changes in meal habits and snacking. They may be very obstinate, refusing to walk and wishing to be carried. Parents may have to give in at times (to avoid the embarrassment of temper tantrums in supermarkets for example) but should not give up trying to implement healthy eating and activity.

- Remember that if children are in real need of food they will eat whatever is available. Food refusal is a luxury and should not result in supplementation.
- Be positive about cooperative behaviour but avoid food rewards.

Action to control weight gain in the very young child can be explained to the children and in some cases they will attempt to follow the advice with vigour. But to follow advice they must have parents who facilitate this by both creating the mealtimes and dietary changes which reduce energy intakes and by giving them opportunities for activity. Children should be encouraged to try to dress themselves, help with simple domestic tasks, show involvement in games, and to socialize both within and outside their families so they do not spend long periods sedentary and bored in front of television or games screen. Helping around the house and garden can be done in a balanced fashion – we are not encouraging children to be drudges but rather to become children with a sense of being involved members of the family unit. Raising the metabolic rate only slightly above resting rates by multiple short periods of activity could be as beneficial to increasing total energy expenditure as short periods of vigorous exercise. Acquiring simple skills and achieving tasks could improve children's self-esteem and self-confidence. If the activities involve helping family members, they could also lead to greater consideration of the needs of others – itself a worthwhile achievement.

Food and love

Weight control will almost certainly involve some aspect of dietary change and probably necessitate some restrictions on what may be favourite foods. When offering advice to parents it is worthwhile recalling the significant place food has in most parent–child relationships, especially mother–child relationships. It is not easy for a mother to deny her child food or to disregard constant nagging for foods as she takes her young child shopping. At much older ages food remains significant in the relationship. It may even be the way a mother who is not good at showing love expresses the bond with her child. Weight management has to work against this natural expression of love and instinctive nurturing.

Sometimes it is grandparents who find it most difficult to control their longing to provide the child with edible treats. Perhaps they do not have quite the same concern for the difficulty of enabling the child to control weight gain since they may not see the child very often. They may view the overweight child positively as 'so like his father' for example. Or if they have hard times when they were bringing up children they may see an overweight child as a healthy child. It is important that all members of the extended family understand the importance of supporting action to help the overweight child and the family develop a healthy lifestyle.

Of course some grandparents are the family members who are most active and concerned about overweight in the grandchildren. They may be very helpful and constructive but sometimes unhelpfully critical and nagging (e.g.:'You shouldn't let her have that'). We should not generalize – supportive grandparents can be very helpful to mothers exhausted by 'taking a strong line' with determined youngsters over food.

Children with disability

Children with disability are more prone to obesity for a variety of reasons. We have already mentioned children with mild learning difficulties who are failing at school, have difficulty with peer relationships and may console themselves with food and isolation. Children who have physical disability may be unable to take part in normal childhood activities and thus have less opportunity to burn off energy than normal children. For some disabled, such as those with hypertonic cerebral palsy, the effort and energy required to perform movements or the difficulties they have eating may mean that they are more likely to be underweight than overweight. So the risk for obesity as a direct consequence of disability is very individual but advice on the management of feeding difficulties, behavioural problems and nutrition can be important in helping to avoid overweight in those children, such as those with Down syndrome, at particular risk (Pipes and Holm 1980).

There are indirect risks for obesity common to many disabilities. Relatives and friends are likely to view disabled children with great sympathy or even a sense of guilt. Such sympathy can translate into overindulgence of the children with sweets and snacks and foods they enjoy. There may be little effort made to encourage the child to eat 'healthy' foods such as vegetables particularly if the disability is associated with feeding difficulties. Similarly, if disabled children are reluctant to be active – something which may be difficult and burdensome – parents and teachers may decide it is easier and less confrontational for the children to be carried, pushed or taken by car when they could actually walk with support or walking aids. In the long term, disabled children are unlikely to benefit from families and friends who neither present them with challenges nor encourage them to develop normal, interpersonal skills which do not centre entirely around themselves.

When a child is diagnosed with disability, advice on a healthy diet and lifestyle for that child should be part of the many discussions the parents will need. Children should be treated as normally as possible in terms of what is expected as good behaviour. Where there is disability which impairs mobility and activity, guidance on controlling energy intakes should be included in early advice. Children who have disorders of growth are at some risk of developing obesity because less energy is utilized in growth. This is particularly true for children with hypothyroidism and growth hormone deficiency because of the lipogenic effects of the hormone deficiencies. However both these hormonal conditions are amenable to treatment so the low energy requirements should not persist once diagnosis has been made. After the first 6 months of life the proportion of total daily energy requirement deposited in tissue growth is $<5\%$ (Widdowson 1971) so children with other growth disturbances, although subjected to some increased risk of obesity, are not inevitably overweight.

Adolescents

We have discussed some issues around changing behaviour in adolescence in earlier chapters. The age is complicated by the physiological changes of adolescence which make it difficult to judge absolute needs in terms of food against the perceived needs of hungry young teenagers surrounded by snacking peers. Telling adolescents what to do can be counterproductive but letting adolescents discuss their lifestyles and where they could make positive changes towards healthier habits with food and exercise may automatically lead to more balanced energy intakes and expenditures (Wilkes and Anderson 2000). Adolescents are still very often dependent on parents for their meals, the food available in their homes and for money to pursue leisure activities. However, when encouraged in the right way, they can integrate taking responsibility for this aspect of themselves as part of their growing independence (particularly if the family have unhelpful eating and activity behaviour).

Adolescence is associated with changed biological timing of sleep (Carskadon *et al.* 2004; Taheri 2006). These young people go to bed later but may actually need more total sleep than immediately prior to adolescence. On school days this may be difficult to achieve so sleep deprivation may be a problem and the typical adolescent behaviour of staying in bed all morning at weekends should probably be accepted – within reason. If the lie-in is very long the circadian clock may be affected and the adolescent may find getting to sleep at night difficult.

Health care professionals will achieve most by listening, making suggestions of what might change in the adolescents' lives as appropriate or when requested but leaving the young person to decide what weight controlling targets, if any, to pursue. Discussing change with adolescents by themselves, although reporting back to the parents the gist of what has been discussed, may give overweight adolescents confidence that the decisions on change are theirs and therefore to be attempted. The decisions for change are not imposed on them by adults and thus for rejection.

Recommendations

- Effective weight control will almost certainly demand some participation in behavioural change by affected children's families. The extended family – aunts and uncles and grandparents – needs to be engaged in the creation of dietary control.

- Whilst changes in energy intakes and expenditures are fundamental to controlling weight, there is potential for influence on weight by promoting 'a good night's sleep', coolish environments and, most significantly, planned television viewing.
- Anticipating the problems that may arise with preschool children, children with disability and adolescents, may help HCPs advise more effectively on weight management.
- The fact that particular behaviours serve roles and purposes for the individuals practising them needs acknowledging. Behavioural change can be difficult to achieve because of the need to fulfil these roles and purposes. Facilitating behavioural change is easier if more beneficial behaviours can be suggested as alternatives to what child or family currently practise.

9

How can we reduce energy intake?

In the previous chapter we discussed general changes in lifestyle which might facilitate the weight control process for overweight and obese children. This chapter deals with creating sustainable changes in energy intakes.

Overweight and obese children do not necessarily have higher energy intakes than the normal weight. Nevertheless overweight/obesity must reflect energy intakes which have been in excess of energy needs for affected individuals. If we are to help these children we need to provide advice on lowering energy intakes which is implementable and sustainable. This involves knowing the 'normal' eating habits of affected children and their families.

How do we find out what overweight/obese children are eating?

Table 9.1 lists methods that can be used to determine energy intakes in individuals under a variety of circumstances and for a variety of purposes. Diet diaries, asking the children or their parents to document on consumption all food and drink taken over a certain period (one day, one week) can be used but, in our experience, compliance is often too poor to be helpful. Retrospective 24-hour recall is the most useful way of making some sort of dietary assessment in the clinic. Details of foods, their preparation, the frequency of consumption and the pattern of meals, snacks, incidental eating and drinking, create understanding of what, where, when and why the subject eats. The aim is to develop a description of foods eaten and the quantities eaten but not a precise, or even estimated, energy intake.

Twenty-four-hour dietary recall/typical day's diet

The purpose is to develop a description of the diet over exactly 24 hours – the previous 24 hours or previous day. The questioner and child (or parent if the

Table 9.1. Methods of assessing dietary energy intakes in individuals

Method	Purpose	Description	'Pros' and 'cons'
Prospective assessments			
Duplicate diet	Precise nutrient intake Research circumstances	Duplicate of everything consumed saved for nutrient analysis	Precise, expensive Impractical outside home or research/metabolic study centre Diet may be altered for convenience or to produce good impression if diet determined by the subject Clinically impractical
Weighed inventory	Precise Used widely in research so inter-study comparisons can be made Similar inventory can be made using household measures rather than weighing the foods but this is less accurate and precise	Weight of all foods and snacks recorded Weight of leftovers subtracted: plate weighed empty then weighed again as foods added; remainders weighed or estimated	Tedious: subjects may omit weighing some foods Subject needs to be familiar with use of scales, recording data, understanding process of weighing plate and then meal items Impractical outside the home Highly likely to choose diet that makes it easier to weigh food or that gives good impression Clinically impractical

Table 9.1. (*cont.*)

Method	Purpose	Description	'Pros' and 'cons'
Retrospective assessments			
24-hour recall	Quite quick method of obtaining an outline of subject's diet Useful guide to a diet in clinical situations	Subject is asked to record all food/snacks/drinks consumed over the past 24 hours Can be augmented with a multi-pass recall which may be more informative	Can be used in the clinic Relatively quick and informative Subjects forget or deliberately overlook some items or may, deliberately or not, include items which have not been consumed Imprecise Gives an idea of the daily diet especially if combined with elements of typical day's diet questionnaire and FFQ
Typical day's diet	Clinically practical Similar to 24-hour dietary recall but avoids limitations of previous 24 hours being atypical	Subject describes meals and snacks consumed on a typical day; this can be done by asking how 24-hour recall differs from the typical day and what variations are there on foods consumed at a particular meal or snack	Can be used in clinical situation Takes longer than 24-hour recall to record Biased towards the impression the subject may wish to give Allows opportunity to explore differences in diet at weekends and (school) holidays Not accurate or precise Provides a good overview on which to give dietary advice
Food frequency questionnaire (FFQ)	Clinically useful in amplifying other retrospective methods although can be quite time consuming	Subject is asked how often per day, week or month particular foods are eaten and usual quantity eaten, method of cooking/preparation if relevant	Used to assess intakes of staples (bread, pasta, rice, potatoes); high energy snacks; junk foods Can use formal, tabulated, recording of items (see Table 9.3) or just pose questions to amplify information from 24-hour recall and typical intake questions

child is too young to comply) work through a day's diet using simple household measures or familiar commercial packaging for quantitative assessment. Cooking methods and outline recipes are needed to provide a concept of the energy density of a food and to facilitate appropriate ideas for dietary change later in the interview. Lunch at school, whether provided by the school, brought from home or bought in a local shop, needs careful itemization. Specific questions also need to be asked about how diets differ over weekends and during school holidays (Turconi *et al.* 2003; Lanigan *et al.* 2004).

Since 24-hour recall may miss some frequent and relevant items (or may be atypical if the previous day was a Sunday for example) it can be amplified by asking how it differs from a typical day's diet: the 'usual' diet. The 'multi-pass' 24-hour recall is also thought to yield more accurate responses than a straight 24-hour recall (Reilly *et al.* 2001). In the multi-pass 24-hour recall, a quick uninterrupted (although prompting and guidance is often necessary with children) recall is run through and this is then followed by discussion of the items recalled and then a review with the subject of the final record. Using a food frequency questionnaire (FFQ) in discussion of the record can enable the subject to remember foods previously omitted (Cade *et al.* 2002).

Food frequency questionnaire

At the end of each account, specific questions are directed at the frequency of consumption of snack items and staple foods since modifying the intakes of these may be a major part of dietary recommendations. Table 9.2 outlines how the FFQ can be recorded formally.

Interpreting the dietary history

Obtaining a good dietary history takes time and patience. There may be a need to probe (verbally) for food items which have been forgotten or carefully ignored. Some families are in a state of denial about the extent to which their children snack. Others seem to regard drinks and foods consumed outside mealtimes or outside home as irrelevant to total energy intake and therefore not worth mentioning. Attempts to explore possible gaps in a typical day's recall may be greeted with defensive responses such as the child 'eats nothing' and 'I told you she eats nothing, nothing for breakfast ....' A follow-up remark such as 'When she has "nothing" for breakfast, what do you give her to eat?' can bring out useful information such as 'Well, she must have something, mustn't she, so I tell her to take some biscuits instead ....'

Avoid seeming judgemental when obtaining a dietary history. Embarrassment in child or family may lead to foods being omitted from the recall and even reluctance to cooperate further if parents feel they are being

Table 9.2. Items to be considered in food frequency questionnaires with some examples of amplification

Item	How many times is item consumed?			Usual size of serving?	Form in which consumed (some suggested questions)
	Per day?[a]	Per week?	Per month?		
Bread				Number of slices	With butter/margarine? White or wholemeal?
Potatoes				Size of potato, number of pieces	How cooked: chipped? fried? Mashed – with milk or butter?
Rice					
Pasta					
Biscuits					What sort of biscuit?
Cakes/buns					Description of form or brand
Chocolate bars					Make, brand, size of bar?
Other confectionery					
Savoury snacks					Packet size? Brand?
Nuts					
Ice cream				Number of scoops? Number of tubs or bars?	
Smoothies					Brand? Sugar free version?
Canned drinks					Sugar free or not?
Whole fruit drinks					

[a] Items could be listed as per each day of week if weekends are very different from schooldays.

criticized or having to confabulate in front of their children. Sometimes parent and child argue over what has been eaten. In such circumstances it may be best to note there is disagreement (which may presage future difficulties when trying to advise and support the family) rather than continue to attempt to discern 'the truth'.

What does the child not eat?

Everyone is entitled to have food preferences with some foods they really do not like. However many overweight and obese children (and some normal weight children) eat a depressingly narrow range of foods. Many seem particularly reluctant to eat vegetables (especially green vegetables), unprocessed meats, fish except when deep fried in batter, fruit other than bananas except as juice or 'smoothies', unsugared cereals, wholemeal bread and cereals, milk and even potatoes except as chips (French fries) and many other items. Some will not drink water, particularly tap water. Encouraging overweight children to eat more varied diets can be one of the most useful but also most difficult aspects of dietary management.

What does the child drink/not drink?

For many children nowadays, drinks are cans of carbonated brand items (Northstone *et al.* 2002; Petter *et al.* 1995). Are these cans normal or low sugar products? If fruit juices are described, are these 'whole' fruit juice or diluted fruit squash? If the latter, do they have added sugar or are they sugar free/low sugar versions? How many cans or what volumes of juice are drunk each day? (The volumes can be large.) Did drinking low energy products only begin as the appointment for assessment of overweight loomed and so may cease as soon as the session is over? If tea or coffee is drunk, is this sweetened or not? And if milk is drunk, is it full cream, semi-skimmed or skimmed?

Where does eating take place?

The following questions may help explore the eating environment.
- Does the child eat breakfast regularly? If not does s/he have breakfast at school?
- Does eating take place as a family or does the child eat alone?
- When and where are snacks consumed?
- Does the child spend much time alone or with friends in his/her room? Does snacking take place then? (Empty crisp packets under the bed?)
- Are foods bought and consumed on the way to and from school or in the lunch break?

At the end of all this dietary questioning it should be possible to answer:
- *What* does the child *eat?*
- *What* does the child *not* eat?
- *What* does the child *drink?*
- *What* does the child *not* drink?

and
- *Why* does the child eat/drink?
- *When* does the child eat/drink?
- *Where* and *with whom* does the child eat/drink?

Attitudes to dietary change

All this information provides the material with which to advise implementable and sustainable dietary change for this child and family. However, child, family and health care professionals need to recognize that weight control is not going to be easy in the profoundly obesogenic modern environment. Dietary change will involve some reduction in energy intake. Reducing the energy intake particularly if the energy expenditure is increased, in effect starves the body. Physiology is likely to rebel at this. Thus none of us adapts readily to a lifestyle which aims to create the negative energy balance needed for weight control and fat loss. We should not criticize the obese for finding this difficult.

Table 9.3 lists societal changes which may have contributed to the burgeoning of overweight amongst children in Britain over recent decades. Most trends are probably not reversible by families but facing up to the effect they have on family eating dynamics can be useful when planning lifestyle changes to reduce energy intakes.

Working mothers have reason to be grateful for the wide range of easy to prepare, oven-ready and ready-to-eat foods now available. However, many of these quick meals have innate problems which make them unhelpful in weight control. Table 9.4 (p. 116) lists some of these disadvantages. It may be helpful for weight control if parents use these meals infrequently and for specific reasons (e.g. genuine hurry to give one child a meal) rather than as a regular way of giving meals – perhaps different for each – to children. Mamun *et al.* (2005) showed that where mothers had a positive attitude towards the family eating together, even if this was not always achieved, overweight was less likely amongst the adolescent children.

The amount adults eat at a meal seems to relate to the numbers with whom they eat – more people, more food – but this does not seem to result in greater total intakes over a period of time, possibly because snacking is less after a good meal in pleasant company (de Castro 1996). A recent study suggests that children also eat more when eating in company of many others (Lumeng & Hillman 2007). It is not clear if this leads (in contrast to the adult

Table 9.3. Societal changes in eating which contribute to the obesity epidemic

Place of meal consumption
- meals are less commonly eaten as a family around a table
- eating in front of the television, alone or as a family, discourages awareness of eating, socializing and, as a result, gives little satisfaction
- decline in school dinner consumption due to cost and perceived poor value of meals offered

Concept of what constitutes a meal
- decline in consumption of breakfast
- choice seen as paramount: separate meals for each member of the family encourages reliance on (energy dense) ready-to-eat or oven-ready meals or quick preparations such as deep frying
- fewer 'meat and two veg.' meals which offer a variety of foods, some of which – the vegetables – are filling but not fattening
- commercially prepared foods: swallowed without much chewing thus reducing chances of satiety

Plethora of snacks
- widely available, relatively cheap and enormously varied
- snack foods are generally energy dense
- increased portion sizes particularly apparent with snack items
- children have more pocket money than in the past
- the variety of forms, flavours and packaging of many snacks contributes to their attraction
- children are surrounded by advertising promoting consumption of certain foods
- advertising pressure and peer pressure encourage consumption even when not hungry
- failure to eat breakfast at home or to eat school dinner may lead to snacking on the way to school
- the decline in some 'traditional' values such as 'don't eat in the street' allows more snacking

findings), to overall higher energy intake over time or is just event related. However the study suggests that eating in an overstimulated, busy and chaotic environment may contribute to excessive energy intakes. Eating as a family at home may be more conducive to balancing energy intakes with energy needs than eating with friends or family in a fast food outlet.

Practical points to suggest to parents and children which may help them plan healthier eating patterns:
- Where practical, eat as a family. Aim at least for all the children to eat together if the parents are unable or unwilling to eat with them.
- Consider where eating takes place. Dedicate an area for family meals, preferably a set table, thus stressing the importance of the family gathering.

- Make mealtimes enjoyable social experiences as well as occasions for eating. Listen to, and talk with, the children.
- Wherever possible take time over meals. Encourage the rest of the family to wait for the slow eaters to finish. Encourage good table manners and thoughtfulness for the eating habits of others.
- Avoid eating in front of the television. Meals are for intra-family communication, not uncommunicative viewing.
- Discourage eating in bedrooms.
- Formalize snacking to no more than once between meals with snacks of low energy content (see later).

Table 9.4. Disadvantages of ready-made meals for weight control in children

Carers have not prepared the food so have little innate feel for its energy density

Energy density is commonly high with predominantly fat and carbohydrate energy since these help keep prices manageable

Food labelling may provide information on nutrient content but not necessarily in ways whereby the relative energy content of a meal is easily appreciated by the consumer: How much is 100g of this food? How big is a 'portion'? How does GDA[a] relate to my child's needs?

Meals are usually soft, very palatable with little need for chewing; they can be consumed with little effort and thus may result in low satiety

The easy palatability of these foods makes them very suitable for eating in front of the television again reducing potential satiety

One or two portion packaging can lead to individual meal consumption with possible reduction of the social interaction gained at family mealtimes

The similarity in presentation and overall texture of different meals seems unlikely to encourage adventurous eating

[a] GDA: Guideline Daily Amount – for explanation see text.

Specific actions to reduce energy intakes

Energy intakes may be reduced by a few generic changes to meal planning:
- Make changes which maximize enjoyment and satisfaction from the modified meals: eat as a family when possible.
- Organize meals and snacks: encourage drinking water but confine eating and other drinking to specified meals and snacks: three main meals and two to three snacks depending on age and family meal structure.
- Manage food refusal.
- Modify fluid intakes with meals and snacks so drinks have minimal energy content.

- Modify food intakes at meals and snacks to provide volume but reduced energy content.
- Use smaller plate sizes.

Dietary modification needs to prioritize changes which can be made by substituting less energy dense foods or foods cooked in ways which do not add to their energy content. This avoids necessarily decreasing the volumes of food offered – although some reduction in the frequency of snacking is almost essential for those overweight children accustomed to heavy snacking. Ideally a weight controlling diet will involve some elements of reduced energy density to the diet and less food/smaller portion sizes (Rolls *et al.* 2006).

We have tabulated many points as we hope this presentation will focus on the varied issues when trying to modify children's diets. Aiming to implement all these changes after the first attendance for weight control advice is unlikely to succeed. Try to get children and families to choose one or two changes to implement on the first occasion they are advised and then follow these changes up with further changes when the children are next seen. Ideally such changes should be fairly general. For example, a child could decide to stop eating 'crisps' and other packet savoury snacks and mother could decide to stop both frying foods and adding fat to grilled food and cooked vegetables. Just avoiding frying one particular food is less likely to be significantly effective – although any change is better than no change and the HCP working with the family is best placed to know what a particular family and child are likely to achieve. Control of weight gain, of fatness or BMI may not be obvious at follow-up if only a few small changes in habits are made but the changes may be sustainable leading to effective weight change and improved health in the future. Families need to be warned that weight change may not be obvious in the early part of the weight controlling activity since they probably have high expectations that their great efforts will be rewarded with immediate very positive change in BMI and weight. They need to understand the gradual build-up to healthy living and the slow nature of successful weight management.

Make changes to maximize enjoyment and satisfaction from meals

One of the reasons dietary management of obesity often fails is that diets recommended are not 'satisfying'. Satisfaction has a number of facets only one of which is physiological satiety. In westernized societies it is relatively rare for us to eat because we are significantly hungry. We eat because food is available, others are eating, it is a certain time of day, we are uncertain when we shall next eat a meal so we snack now just in case that meal never comes, we are celebrating with friends, we feel the need to cheer ourselves up or to reward ourselves etc. Creating strategies to reduce the desire to eat when there is no physiological need is crucial for effective obesity management programmes. Potential 'temptations' need to be minimized and psychological satiety maximized.

Organize meals and snacks

It is impossible to give a specific timetable of meals and snacks for obese children since what is practical will depend on family issues and what is needed will depend on the age, sex and individual lifestyle of the child. Eating should be planned around three main meals which should include breakfast. Snacks should be planned if there is a long period between meals. It may be more tactical to provide snack time closer to the meal that is past rather than the meal that is to come. Lack of appetite due to recent snacking could lead to food refusal at the mealtime followed by hunger later – leading to more snacking. This is particularly likely with young children whose stomachs are relatively small and who can easily feel sated with drinks or confectionery snacks. As total contrast, adolescent boys going through their growth spurt and staying up late in the evenings may need substantial snacks pre-bedtime.

Deal with boredom and hunger

'I'm bored' is often a reason for children to demand food or to snack. Most of us find that if our minds are fully occupied and we are active and busy we do not have the same need to eat as when we are relaxed. Widening children's interests and involving them in hobbies, preferably but not essentially those requiring expenditure of activity, can be helpful in reducing the number of occasions when children think of seeking food.

If items such as biscuits, sweets and crisps are not in the house this should reduce both 'temptation' and opportunity to eat these. Making snack foods less available requires cooperation from the whole family and not just the overweight child. As far as possible parents should make decisions about where change should come in collaboration with their children but this will depend on the age of family members. Schools in Britain have recently been made to alter what is available at many of their food outlets, with the aim of making high energy snacks less available during school hours. The effects of these changes have yet to be determined. Children may simply alter their habits and seek the snacks outside school during breaks rather than restrict themselves to what is on offer in school. Parents at home (and the teachers in school) need to supplement change with discussion on the reasons for the change with the children.

The role of foods with low glycaemic index

The glycaemic index (GI) of a food is a reflection of the 'area under the curve' of the blood glucose response compared with that of a 'standard' meal. Foods which produce lower glycaemic responses may be more satiating (Warren *et al.* 2003) since the gradual insulin response is less likely to be followed by the dramatic reactive fall in glucose which may induce hunger or 'dumping' symptoms and a need to eat. The 'area under the curve' does not indicate the rate of rise in blood glucose. Slow rise and fall may produce a similar total GI as a rapid rise and rapid fall but with a very different insulin response and different effect on blood glucose changes. However, it is thought by some that foods with high GI and high sugar content encourage overeating because of the dramatic rebound fall in blood glucose. Certainly they seem to create less short-term satiety (Alvina and Araya 2004). This provides another reason for avoiding energy dense snacks particularly those high in sugars (Ludwig 2007).

In practice food GIs vary quite widely between individuals. The lists of foods of high, medium and low GI seem very mixed and sometimes rather puzzling. Why should jacket potato have a high GI and boiled potato a medium GI? Foods with high fibre content are mostly of lower GI than those with refined carbohydrate. It is difficult to plan diets on the basis of choosing low GI foods because speculating correctly on a food's GI grouping is not easy. Moreover it is the overall (carbohydrate) energy rather than the glucose level reached which makes most contribution to weight control. Rather than worry about foods' GI values it may be simpler, as a general policy, to aim to include as many foods that are 'whole foods' or high fibre foods with relatively low energy content in the weight control diet (Augustin *et al.* 2002). Whole foods and high fibre cereals may be less rapidly consumable, but, because of the fibre content, they may seem more filling (Santangelo *et al.* 1998). The fibre content can also make them less energy dense.

Manage food refusal

Everyone is entitled to personal dislikes in foods (e.g. custard, mayonnaise, marmalade, liver). Such dislikes can be respected by preparing meals where particular foods do not have to be put on the plate. But an environment in which, with minor exceptions, the family eats the meal provided and expects no alternative is highly desirable. Eating along with the family may encourage younger children to eat foods that are usually refused rather as such children sometimes 'learn' to like these foods (or sometimes learn to dislike) when eating with peers at school dinners. From time to time children are confronted by foods which are not their favourite but are 'on the menu' and which are expected to be consumed. A tactic of 'It's there so eat it up' is likely to fail if one of both parents refuses the same items. If you want your children to eat vegetables, start by enjoying them yourselves (Cooke *et al.* 2004).

Altering the habits of choosey children through the 'There is no alternative' approach will not always be effective. If the food is not eaten, even after gentle encouragement, parent or carer should avoid complaining or trying to force the child to eat. These will only reinforce food refusal particularly amongst older children. No comment or an expression of slight disappointment that the food is uneaten is probably best. A preferred food should not be offered as alternative. Foods refused without good reason should be offered on future occasions. Infants and toddlers may take 10 to 20 tastings before they find some foods acceptable (Wardle *et al.* 2003). Families who give up easily when confronted by food refusal may find their children habitually consume diets that are very restricted in variety and often energy dense (Birch and Fisher 1998).

Principles of developing diets that are varied in taste and texture:

- Encourage introduction of foods at weaning which require chewing.
- Encourage consumption of whole fruits and vegetables rather than pureed or juiced products.
- Encourage cooking using basic ingredients. This may require cookery education for families.
- Build up knowledge about the relative energy content of different foods and different cooking methods.
- Respect children's specific likes and dislikes but teach children that the consequence of not eating foods is going without. Food refusal is not 'rewarded' by a favourite food as an alternative.
- Promote enjoyable eating as a family group.
- Encourage a sense of adventure with tactical introduction of new foods and new ways of preparing foods, particularly through using whole foods more.

Manage fluid intakes

The choice in fluids now available to children is enormous even in low income countries. Drinking with meals may reduce food intake. Drinking interrupts and therefore slows the process of eating. Water, even bottled water, has no energy content and is thus eminently suitable for consumption with meals. However water is not a popular drink with many British children. Concerns about the processes water supplies now go through before reaching the kitchen tap may account for some of the decline in tap water drinking in UK homes.

Why is so much attention focused on the role of commercial drinks in the epidemic of obesity in today's children? Several studies from the UK and elsewhere relate soft drink consumption with obesity and reduced soft drink consumption with improved weight status (James *et al.* 2004). Most commercial soft drinks contain large amounts of sugar and thus energy. They have few other nutrients and little satiety effect. Even if the drinks are 'low energy', they are very sweet possibly encouraging 'a sweet tooth' and a desire for more drinks of this kind (which may not always be low energy versions) (Petter *et al.* 1995). Some sweeteners, such as sorbitol, cause loose stools and contribute to 'toddler diarrhoea'.

'Fresh' fruit juices sold in cartons are promoted as 'healthy' because they are sources of vitamin C and vitamin A. For obese children use should be confined to aperitifs, for example starters at breakfast time, rather than as means of quenching thirst. One 180-ml glass of orange juice may contain 290 kJ (68 kcals). One whole orange contains around 226 kJ (52 kcals) and takes much longer to consume.

The following are some points relevant to reducing the energy intake from drinks:

- Avoid or minimize use of commercial carbonated drinks. Do not use to quench thirst.
- Pour bottled/canned drinks into a cup or mug and do not necessarily offer the whole can/bottle to one child.
- If carbonated drinks are deemed necessary from time to time, use the reduced energy forms but keep intakes to low volumes.
- Keep drinks of whole fruit juice to small amounts (cup or small glass) offered at the beginning of meals such as breakfast. Do not use to quench thirst.
- If children are reluctant to drink plain water with their meals use bottled water if this is affordable. Encourage older children to drink tap or bottled water in preference to other commercial drinks. (Water bottles appear the same when refilled from the tap.)
- If children refuse to drink water in any form, use fruit squashes which require dilution. Make them up in very dilute form. Preferably use sugar free versions (this does not discourage liking of sweetness in drinks but does diminish the energy intake from the drinks).
- When children drink tea or coffee or other hot beverages, do not add sugar to the drinks. Avoid use of artificial sweeteners in drinks since these may only encourage a desire for sweetness.

Most commercial drink dispensers have now been removed from schools and replaced by water dispensers or occasionally fruit juice dispensers. Some schools issue children with bottles of water at the beginning of each term. The children are encouraged to refill these as necessary from drinking water sources around their school. This seems a sensible practice which fits in with the current young culture of clutching a bottle of water at all times and in all places.

Modify food energy density

There are three main approaches, which should be combined, to reducing energy intakes without making it obvious to the subject that they are consuming less:

- Use cooking methods that add less energy to foods.
- Change to low energy versions of foods.

- Change the balance of foods on the plate (Figure 9.1): one half of the plate is fruit or vegetables, one quarter meat/fish/eggs or other protein source and one quarter staple of potatoes, rice, pasta or bread.

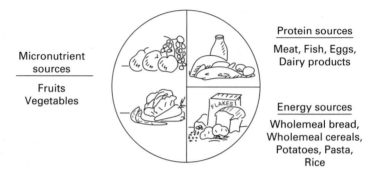

Micronutrient
sources
_____

Fruits
Vegetables

Protein sources
_____

Meat, Fish, Eggs,
Dairy products

Energy sources
_____

Wholemeal bread,
Wholemeal cereals,
Potatoes, Pasta,
Rice

Figure 9.1 The balance of foods in the weight control meal

Table 9.5 suggests how cooking and food presentation strategies can reduce the energy content of meals without making the reduction in energy intakes obvious. Changing standard foods to low energy versions (see Table 9.6) can also disguise the lower energy intakes.

Table 9.5. Structural changes to diets and eating which may help control weight in the overweight and obese

Cook at home as much as possible so the composition of the meal is known and can be adjusted for weight control

Use commercial low energy versions of products which are eaten regularly (Table 9.6)

Alter the way foods are prepared to reduce their energy content; for example, eat potatoes boiled or baked rather than as chips

Cut out added fats in cooking. Do not add butter to vegetables or potatoes on serving. Grill (without added fat) or boil or microwave rather than fry. Roast meats without adding fat

Offer foods in forms which may be more satiating, such as wholemeal breads and cereals and whole fruits

Reduce quantity of foods with high energy density but little contribution either to satiety or breadth of nutrient intake: butter/margarine and other fats, sugar, sweets

Alter the proportion of foods on the plate: larger portions of vegetables, smaller portions of meat and staple

Present meals on smaller plates to reduce the volume of food subtly

The single focus diets so popular with the media and 'slimming' magazines make recommendations on specific food groups (e.g. low carbohydrate or high protein diets) which are often unsuitable for children who, because of

Table 9.6. Some useful low energy versions of foods

Semi-skimmed or skimmed milk^a

Low energy spreads on bread (these have the advantage of being spreadable straight from the refrigerator unlike butter)

Low energy bread

Breakfast cereals which are not sugar coated, frosted or with added fruit and which preferably have relatively unrefined cereal and which are served without added sugar

Low energy yogurts (not all 'low fat' yogurts are low energy so study the nutrition information carefully)

Sugar free fruit squashes which require dilution

Low energy slimmers' soups – but it is probably more satisfactory to prepare home-made thin soups if this can be done

Leaner cuts of meat or meat with the fat cut off; reduced fat sausages, minced meat

---

^{a} Semi-skimmed and skimmed milk are not recommended in UK as drinks for children under 5 years old although, if the children are on 'balanced diets', semi-skimmed milk may be given to children over 2 years old. For children under 2 who are overweight but eating a varied diet, semi-skimmed milk is probably appropriate provided there is clinical supervision of progress.

growth and development, need 'balanced' diets with good sources of protein, essential fatty acids and micronutrients even if their weight demands reduced energy (Adam-Perrot *et al.* 2006). Diets that focus on reduction of one nutrient type provide no guidance for the sustainable eating habits which would allow weight maintenance once weight control has been achieved. Working with child and family to outline a diet which suits their usual eating pattern and as far as possible meal content allows opportunities to ensure a variety of nutrients in the diet.

Providing specific advice

Some children and families want diet sheets which list what they should eat and when. They feel they can follow these with confidence (but not necessarily success). Diet sheets need to be developed individually for each overweight child or adolescent and his/her family. Such a diet sheet can be developed by going through the typical day's diet determined at the beginning of the interview and indicating where and how changes can be made. In terms of developing sustainability it is vital that families are not just told what to eat but are given food focused dietary advice (Gehling *et al.* 2005). They learn which foods are high in energy and possibly not necessary, which foods children need but in reduced amounts and which foods can be eaten in abundance. One approach to dieting which teaches this with some success is the Traffic Light Diet (TLD) approach (Epstein *et al.* 1985, 1998).

Table 9.7. Traffic Light Diet management of weight control

Colour code for food	Types of food included[a]	Freedom of consumption
Red	Confectionery, crisps, chips, takeaways, canned drinks, fried foods, ice cream	No more than once or twice a week but preferably avoided altogether for overweight/obese
Amber	Meat, fish, staples, dairy products	Quantity of these foods should be controlled and regulated
Green	Whole fruit and vegetables	At least five portions a day as per UK government guidelines but quantities consumed need not be restricted[b]

[a] Items that we feel should be categorized here.

[b] Bananas, whilst having many of the benefits of other fruits, do provide significant contribution to energy because of their size: consumption should perhaps be in the 'Amber' category. Avocados are also energy dense but are less likely to be consumed excessively in the UK. Any fruit if eaten to excess can create significant energy intake but is likely to be fairly satiating and thus helpful in dieting.

Here foods are divided into red, amber and green categories. The colour category determines how much these foods should feature in the overweight/obese child's diet. Table 9.7 summarizes the main principles of the diet. Lists of foods falling into each colour category can be obtained commercially but the principal of TLD can be applied to a particular child's diet without significant nutrition specialist involvement. Table 9.8 lists some 'red' foods which should be avoided as much as possible. The foods in Table 9.6 can be included as 'amber' foods: useful components of the diet but to be consumed in moderation.

Food labelling

One of our concerns about recommending the TLD is that the family may get confused messages due to the new Traffic Signal labelling of foods recently adopted by the Food Standards Agency (FSA) and some supermarkets (Figure 9.2). In the TLD foods are described as red (avoid), amber (eat in modest amounts) or green (eat as much as you like) according to their overall energy content and energy density and portion size. High fat or high sugar/carbohydrate content are likely to be associated with red foods.

In the traffic *signalling* approach to food *labelling*, foods are graded red, amber or green for four nutrients. Thus a food may be red for fat content

Table 9.8. Foods that should be consumed only infrequently, if at all, and in no more than small quantities[a]

Sweets, chocolate
Chips, crisps, savoury snacks, nuts
Carbonated drinks, fruit juices, sweetened fruit squashes
Buns, biscuits, cakes, puddings, jams, syrup, honey
Fried foods
Hamburgers, sausages, patés
Salad dressings and mayonnaise
Vegetables with oils or butter added in presentation
Tinned fruits in syrup
Custards, sauces, thickened gravy
Cream, fromage frais, yogurt, cheese

[a] Some of these items can be replaced by low energy versions (see Table 9.6).

because it is high in fat (and thus high in energy also) but may also carry amber or green labels if there is not much saturated fat, little sugar and/or salt content is low. Asking the busy parent to sort out the foods that are red in terms of fats or sugars versus those red for salt or saturated fats but not for overall fat and sugar content seems to be asking quite a lot of the average consumer. However there have been appreciative responses to the labelling system from a variety of non-governmental, including women's,

	Solids g/100 g			Liquids g/100 ml			Items >250g g/portion
	Low (green)	Medium (amber)	High (red)	Low (green)	Medium (amber)	High (red)	High (red)
FAT	<3	3–20	>20	<1.5	1.5–10	>10	>21
SATURATES	<1.5	1.5–5	>5	<0.75	0.75–2.5	>2.5	>6
SUGAR	<5	5–15	>15	<2.5	2.5–7.5	>7.5	>18
SALT	<0.3	0.3–1.5	>1.5	<0.3	0.3–1.5	>1.5	>2.4

Figure 9.2 Traffic signal labelling criteria for categories of food. (Food Standards Agency: www.foodstandards.gov.uk)

organizations. Unfortunately the confusion so familiar in food labelling has not been resolved since not all UK supermarkets have adopted the FSA method. Some are indicating the nutrient content of a food by its percentage of Guideline Daily Amount (%GDA), that is the proportion of the average daily requirement of an adult man for each nutrient mentioned, provided either by 100 g of the food or by the total item. This does not seem an approach which is helpful to parents seeking low energy foods for their overweight children.

We recommend that parents and children have the food labelling alternatives explained to them and are advised that foods which are red for fats and/or sugars are foods which should be consumed infrequently if at all. However mothers should be encouraged to look at the energy (calorie) content of the foods they purchase, noting whether the amount indicated is per portion, per whole or fraction of an item or per 100 g and, at the same time as looking at the food label, note the weight of the whole item. Not easy, but interpretation of food labels can be learnt. Reading food labels should be recommended even if only for the parent or child to bring questions to the clinic at the next attendance.

Sustainability in dietary change

Weight control needs to be something that can be sustained as desired effects on weight will come only slowly. Ideally children learn to live and eat more 'healthily' and sustain this lifestyle into adulthood. Modest rather than dramatically restrictive dietary regimes would seem more likely to be sustainable in the long term. Thus confectionery (mostly TLD 'red' items) consumption could be heavily restricted but not totally eliminated. Money saved not buying 'red' items could be directed towards buying reduced energy versions of other foods since these are sometimes more expensive than their more energy dense 'normal' equivalents. ('Low fat' confectionery is not a good exchange for normal confectionery since fat is often replaced by simple carbohydrates and the energy density may be relatively unaffected. Similarly, 'diabetic' foods are not necessarily low in energy although they are usually low in sugars. Doing without confectionery items altogether seems a wiser policy.)

Whilst not following the TLD recommendations totally, we suggest that foods listed in Table 9.8 are foods that should be eaten very infrequently or not at all. Children and parents may react 'but that leaves nothing to eat'. This is where children with varied tastes and more adventurous eating habits are so much easier to help than those with limited dietary likes but perhaps children in this former group are less likely to get obese in the first place?

As pointed out earlier, the foods listed in Table 9.6 can be substitutes for usual foods which either by energy density or by quantity eaten make significant contributions to children's daily energy intakes. Their substitution leads to lowered energy intake with no change in volume of food eaten.

Lower energy content in a food is not a reason to consume more of that food since that negates the effect of the lowered energy density. These foods are replacements. If they are still fairly energy dense (e.g. reduced fat sausages) because they replace a very energy dense food, consumption should still be infrequent. Further, the method of cooking may be relevant if the food is to retain its lower energy content. Frying, instead of grilling, energy reduced sausages unnecessarily increases energy density and reduces the benefit of the 'low energy' food.

So what is there left to eat?

The foods listed in Table 9.8 may constitute the major part of the diet for some children. The readiness of children and their families to accept substantial changes in the range of foods consumed tests the real ability of children and their carers to control the children's weight. Without some change in eating habits, including changes in the components of meals, it will be very difficult to control weight. The present environment, through effects on both activity and diet, has precipitated the obesity. Without change in this, why should obesity reduce?

For children and families who accept change, a mixed satisfying diet can be relatively easy to devise, although persuading children to forgo the temptations of confectionery, commercial carbonated drinks, fried foods, chips and crisps may pose problems. Table 9.9 outlines the sort of diet children could follow which should ensure reasonable satisfaction and yet be energy reduced. This is a diet probably only achieved after some time as the summation of incremental small changes to the diet. Whether it is ever achieved will probably depend on how effective less substantial changes are in controlling the child's weight. Adolescent boys for example may slim quite readily on diets which are still high in energy compared with those required to control weight in younger children, adolescent girls or adults.

Despite the outline in Table 9.9, it is impossible to develop one recommended diet which applies equally to all children since the age, size, sex and individual requirements of children are such significant determinants of nutritional needs. Table 9.9 is developed with a schoolchild in mind. But the amount of bread (for example) children eat will vary with age as well as family habit. Bread can provide a useful 'filler' particularly for adolescent boys. What is eaten with or on the bread may make a greater contribution to the energy content of the food item than the bread itself. If a child normally consumes four slices of bread a day, it should be reasonable to suggest that three slices a day should be the future maximum. Low energy bread may be

Table 9.9. Outline for possible meal plan[a]

Breakfast	Unsugared cereal, semi-skimmed milk, no sugar. Toast, thin scrape of low energy margarine, small quantity of low sugar jam/marmalade or honey. Apple/orange/other fresh fruit. Semi-skimmed milk, unsweetened tea/coffee to drink
Mid morning	Water/dilute low energy fruit squash/unsweetened coffee/tea and piece of fruit
Lunch[b]	Low energy soup, wholemeal bread roll, small amount of margarine/butter or cold meat/tinned oily fish with oil drained off/small portion of cheese with salad[c] or meat or fish grilled, stewed or roast without added fat, plus good helping of vegetables. No potatoes or small helping of boiled potatoes/pasta/rice if these are not eaten with the evening meal. Fresh fruit
After school	Unsweetened drink, piece of bread, thin scrape low energy margarine and low sugar jam or small amount of honey or small piece of cake or biscuit
Evening meal	Meat or fish cooked to use as little fat as practical, vegetables cooked without adding oil/other fat, pasta/rice/medium sized baked or boiled potatoes without butter/oil added. Fruit stewed without added sugar but using sweetener instead[d]
Before bed	Unsweetened drink. Fruit or small portion of cheese and biscuits preferably without margarine/butter or bowl of unsweetened cereal with semi-skimmed milk

[a] The diet will vary with the age of the child in that small children are likely to eat less in the evening (they should be asleep in bed) and whether there is a snack on return from school will depend on timing of the evening meal etc.
[b] For detailed recommendations for school dinner see text.
[c] Salad implies lettuce, tomatoes, cucumber, peppers, celery etc. preferably without dressing, rather than pasta/corn/beans laced with oil or mayonnaise.
[d] Saccharine can be dissolved in warm water and added after the fruit has been cooked.

an alternative but the slices are usually smaller than the standard loaf slices and may still have toppings which are as energy rich as on normal energy breads.

'I'm hungry'

It is a problem when trying to control children's dietary intakes that demands for food can come at unplanned times. Sometimes this is boredom. Sometimes it is true hunger. Sometimes it is a determination to nag a parent. A first reaction is to reassure the child that the next meal is not far ahead (if true). Then to engage the child in conversation or play or some activity which takes the child's thoughts away from food ('Yes, dear. Why don't you take the

Table 9.10. Possible snacks to offer if child complains of hunger in between snack or meal periods

Drink of water or diluted low energy fruit squash
Cup of unsweetened tea or coffee for older children
Fresh fruit (not bananas or grapes)
Raw carrot and raw celery strips (these suggest very dedicated slimmers!)
Crispbread with very thin scrape of low energy margarine
Slice of wholemeal bread with thin scrape of low energy margarine

dog out for a walk before your tea?'). A drink of water or dilute low energy squash may solve the problem. The items we list as a 'last resort' in Table 9.10 look pretty cruel but the reality is that if all demands for food are met, children and their families will achieve nothing in their efforts to control weight. Adolescent boys at the height of their growth spurt may be reflecting genuine need for more food. Apparent needs require sensitive balancing against what has been eaten over the rest of the day.

School dinners

When children are at school there are limited opportunities to eat. This makes the school day a good time to control energy intakes since children should have their minds occupied by other things during lessons and this may help override the minor hunger or desire for food which can come with boredom. For some children it is easier to achieve weight control during term time than during the holidays for these reasons. Our outline diet is quite restrictive with recommendations for nutrition at school lunchtime. A child who is on free school meals may be reliant on the school dinner for the one 'proper' meal of the day. Thus every child needs to be advised in ways that are appropriate for his or her circumstances.

In the UK the majority of children do not go home for lunch. In the past the chief aim of school dinners apart from feeding the child was to provide good nutrition for children who might not receive adequate food at home. Times have changed and the need now is to help children eat 'healthily' without promoting obesity rather than to prevent malnutrition. Outcry over the quality of school meals in England and Wales has led to a boost in the money available to feed each child but schools are still under a lot of pressure from the government and from the public and the media to improve the nutritional quality of the meals and to make school meals better value for money. This does not necessarily mean that meals are less energy dense but more low energy choices and particularly vegetables, salads and fresh fruit are now available. Many children still prefer to bring packed lunches rather than eat school food. Or they visit local shops to buy snacks – crisps, cola, chocolate bars – for lunch.

What can be done to help children eat weight controlling diets at school? One approach is to support communal meals at school when all participate, even the teachers, regardless of whether lunch comes from home or school. By educating teachers and children about good nutrition, by encouraging children to eat communally and semi-formally, better meal habits may be adopted and the principles of good nutrition imbued (Sahota *et al.* 2001). When lunches are eaten under these circumstances with emphasis on 'healthy' foods, teachers have sometimes commented that the children's behaviour in afternoon lessons has improved. This is a valuable bonus.

What should be eaten? Table 9.9 includes suggestions for schoolchildren trying to control their weight. Cold meats and salad, low energy soup with bread or the meat course from the school dinner with any pastry removed and a good helping of vegetables. Chips and roast potatoes should be avoided. Whether children are offered potatoes or other staple may depend on whether their lunches are their main meal or whether they have a further substantial cooked meal in the evening. A piece of fruit or fresh fruit salad could be offered for dessert whatever is eaten for the first course.

Children bringing packed lunches could bring a box salad with items such as lettuce, tomato, celery, cucumber and a small piece of cheese, slice of cold ham or chicken leg (for example) together with fresh fruit. Alternatively, a small thermos of low energy soup and a bread roll instead with fresh fruit could be provided if parents feel their children must have something hot in the winter. If sandwiches seem the only practical way of producing a packed lunch, these should preferably be wholemeal bread with a thin scraping of low energy spread and ideally a low energy filling such as ricotta (cottage) cheese or lettuce and tomato or a slice of lean ham. Fresh fruit can be included with the lunch.

In this chapter we have been discussing diet. How restrictive a diet needs to be to control weight is dependent on many things other than the individual energy intake. Adolescent boys grow very rapidly. Physiologically their bodies are developing predominantly lean tissue. The tendency is to lose some fat during male puberty. High energy intakes are required to meet these physiological needs. Quite modest energy reduction can lead to very successful weight control in boys in this age group as they 'grow into their weight'. The same is sadly not true for adolescent girls who have shorter and therefore smaller growth spurts, often early in puberty. Further the female body tends to lay down fat more at puberty so the physiological tendency is encouraging obesity. Pubertal girls have great difficulty controlling fat deposition even when they modify their lifestyles effectively. Energy intake from the diet is of course only one aspect of energy balance and as we explained at the beginning of the chapter is dependent on the whole environment in which eating takes place. Without concern for the whole lifestyle which includes how physically active individuals are, a prescription of energy intake for weight control will be an unrealistic and unsustainable aspiration.

Recommendations

- Find out as much as practical about the family and child's normal eating habits.
- Explain that dietary change is not easy: children need role models for eating habits and the whole family is likely to benefit from positive qualitative changes in their diets.
- Recognize that providing high quality diets may be more difficult for some families than others because of poverty, 'food deserts', time available for home cooking, cooking skills within the families etc.
- Where appropriate encourage parents and children to learn to cook.
- Advise on organizing meals and snacks.
- Give families advice on the nutrient content of food items where appropriate and where such advice is likely to be helpful rather than confusing.
- Explain the principles of Traffic Light Diets (TLD).
- Advise on reading and trying to interpret food labels: traffic signalling and GDA.
- Go through the daily diet focusing on foods and helping the family choose strategies for reducing the energy content of the diet without necessarily reducing food volume:
    Use food brands and preparations with lower energy density where possible.
    Use cooking methods which reduce the energy content of the meals.
    Exclude foods on the 'red' list as much as practicable.
- Help children and families choose initial targets for dietary change: e.g. get families, especially children if they are old enough, to participate by setting dietary targets for themselves at the first attendance.
- Advise small incremental changes as a practical policy for effective weight control.
- Help the family and child consider what options are available to them for reducing the energy content of the school lunch.
- Remember that changes which are easy for some are very difficult for others and praise all efforts to make positive change.

10

How can we increase energy expenditure?

Efforts to increase energy expenditure deserve as much emphasis as those to reduce energy intake for the management of overweight/obesity. Yet, in the public mind, management seems dominated by 'dieting'. This is surprising since data suggest that mean energy intakes for UK children under 15 years fell consistently over the latter half of the twentieth century (Gregory *et al.* 1995; Gregory and Lowe 2000). Some decline in energy expenditure as PA must have contributed at least in part to the increased prevalence of obesity. Multi-pronged approaches which include changes to both dietary habits and PA are now widely recognized as the ways to effective management in adults (Chief Medical Officer 2004; Lobstein *et al.* 2004). In children, both increased PA and reduced sedentary behaviour are effective in the treatment and prevention of childhood obesity (Summerbell *et al.* 2003, 2005).

What has changed?

Why has PA declined so much in children of many westernized countries? We list below some of the societal and environmental items which have led to falling PA levels in many present-day societies.

Urbanization

Roads are much busier with traffic than in the past and many play areas and open spaces in towns have been lost. The environment and the perceptions of the environment seem very important to the extent to which children are active outside the home (Davison and Lawson 2006; Evenson *et al.* 2006; Alton *et al.* 2007). Although studies show that children who perceive a lack of parks and play areas near where they live tend to be less active, those who perceive high traffic risk where they walk tend to be those who walk *more*. This might be because the children with high levels of walking, if they walk in congested areas, are more likely to be warned of the risks from traffic than those who are unlikely to walk there anyway. In general it seems that those who enjoy walking and are prepared to walk will walk, whatever the perception of the environment, whereas those who do not enjoy walking will find reason to remain at home (Alton *et al.* 2007).

Transport

Much travel is no longer 'active' travel. The average mileage walked per year by the UK population has declined by 26% in the past 50 years. The distances cycled per year have fallen by 86% over the same period. Cycle mileage by children fell by more than 40% between 1975/6 and 1993/4 (Department for Transport 2002). Currently only 2% of secondary schoolchildren and 1% of primary schoolchildren go to school on their bicycles (Department for Transport 2007). Both car ownership and two-car homes have increased. More than half of the children in the UK are driven to school (Department for Transport 2002).

Security in the community

Concern for children going out unaccompanied by adults relates to both dangers from traffic and fear of undesirable strangers. For parents, perceptions of stranger danger and concern about road traffic make them reluctant to allow their children to play out of doors or walk around the community unsupervised by adults. Alton *et al.* (2007) found 62.8% of children and 76.1% of adults in Birmingham UK were anxious about strangers in the local environment when questioned. Thus it is no surprise that parents fill their homes with entertainments to keep their children safe and indoors despite the social isolation and negative health effects such entertainments may bring.

Smaller homes and gardens

Whilst average housing standards have improved greatly over the past century, many houses have smaller living areas than in the past and, in particular, smaller gardens. Houses are close together and family homes may be apartment blocks. It is more difficult for children to 'let off steam', romp around, or just play vigorously in house, garden or yard without complaints from neighbours and consequent parental embarrassment.

Home equipment

Home management, in which children may have played an active part in the past, is less time and energy consuming because labour-saving devices for homes and gardens are so widespread.

Entertainment

Audiovisual media have created satisfying home-based, sedentary entertainment. In 2002 in the UK 99% of households owned a television. Fifty-two per cent of under-16s, including 36% of preschool children, had a television set in their bedroom. Forty-four per cent of households had access to satellite, cable or digital television.

Educational aspirations

Physical education has not been a priority in schools in the face of pressure to implement the National Curriculum and fulfil educational targets. This situation is beginning to change but the sale of so many school playing-fields towards the end of the last century has made it difficult for some schools to revive games and sports adequately. Public Service Framework targets are for high-quality PE lasting 2 hours a week or more involving 75% of 5–16-year-olds by 2006 and 85% by 2008.

Time

The UK working population has a reputation for long hours. Parents may spend much of the day at work and getting to and from work. They return home tired and possibly unenthusiastic about taking the children for a walk, to the park or simply playing games with the children in the garden – particularly in winter when it is likely to be dark when they get home. (Could abandoning Greenwich Mean Time improve the population's nutritional status?)

Employment

For adults many jobs that were traditionally laborious are much less so because of mechanization. Computers and emails make many work roles more desk-bound than before. Trends have been from laborious industrialized manufacturing jobs to those that are service-based and often less physically demanding.

The complexity of the obesity epidemic

There are many other reasons why children are less active but these examples illustrate how complex are the drivers of the obesity epidemic. Many of the changes we describe cannot be altered by parents keen to improve their children's and perhaps their own activity. However, recognizing what has changed may help people to devise lifestyles that override the effects of change.

The health benefits of activity

Physical activity is beneficial for health independent of the effects it has on control of fatness (Warburton *et al.* 2006a). Low levels of PA increase the risks for coronary heart disease, stroke, type 2 diabetes mellitus, some cancers and many other chronic conditions (Health Survey for England 2004, 2006) independent of any increase in weight. By contrast, increased energy expenditure in PA reduces the risks of these conditions in both obese and normal weight even if it does not reduce weight. The co-morbidities of obesity are more common in overweight adults than in overweight children but, as explained in Chapter 6, more and more overweight/obese adolescents and younger children now present with complications to their overweight. Physical activity also improves musculo-skeletal skills and coordination and enhances cardiorespiratory efficiency in response to exertion – the 'training' effect and one criterion of physical fitness. Weight bearing activity helps minimize the lean body mass (LBM) loss that goes with fat loss (Schwingshandl *et al.* 1999) and promotes bone mineralization and the high peak bone mass in adolescence which protects against osteoporosis later.

Physical activity also promotes psychological well-being and is helpful in the treatment of mild to moderate depression. Many types of activity create opportunities for children to interact through informal play or in formal PE: games or gym classes at school, clubs or any play area. Developing eye–limb co-ordination and learning to cope emotionally with teamwork, winning and losing, are important aspects of childhood development. Even activities practised by a child alone can teach balance, co-ordination, judgement of distance and numerous other physical and social skills. A physically active lifestyle should be started from birth. Sadly, unlike eating, PA is optional in modern society. The sedentary lifestyle is now a viable alternative. So, if PA is beneficial for children but insufficiently practised, how do we assess children's activity levels and what can we do to promote more active lifestyles amongst the overweight and obese?

Assessing levels of activity in children

For most children, energy expenditure in moderate to vigorous activity varies from day to day depending on the weather, the school timetable, whether it is weekday, weekend or holiday. Activity levels also tend to show differences with age and gender. The time spent in PA and the intensity of the PA commonly decline as children grow older. The decline is particularly marked around puberty and more noticeable for pubertal girls. Boys are, on average, more physically active than girls at all ages (Armstrong *et al.* 1990).

Many children are more active on schooldays than at weekends or during the holidays since school provides structured episodes of moderate to vigorous activity in games and gym together with perhaps walking to school and playing games in break periods or after school. Other children are very active after school, at weekends or during the holidays, playing outside, taking part in formal or non-formal games, using sports facilities and swimming pools, taking part in clubs or dancing classes or simply walking or cycling with their families. On the whole children seem more active, and more ready to be active, in summer than in winter.

Assessing activity

Table 10.1 lists some ways of assessing PA in children. Questionnaires of activity and activity diaries are the most immediate ways of assessing activity levels although responses are inevitably very subjective. Few questionnaires are validated and direct questioning may be needed to develop a good picture of children's normal PA. Some adults and children interpret activity as the 'formal' PE of games and gym. Questioning may need to probe for information about less formal episodes of activity (do the children rush around the house after school or sit quietly watching television or, preferably perhaps for parents, something in between?). Questioning also needs to be broad. What is happening when the children are not perceived as being physically active? How sedentary are they and for how long? The massive increase in time spent in sedentary behaviours rather than the decline in PA may have contributed most to the decline in energy expenditure that has helped promote the current epidemic of childhood obesity.

When questioning about the 'usual' PA of overweight/obese children, the aim is not a precise description from which total daily energy expenditure can be calculated but an overall impression of whether the children participate in or avoid games, PE and other opportunities to exercise and whether they are largely sedentary or active at home. Table 10.2 shows the Chief Medical Officer's 2004 recommendations for minimum daily activity of British children and adults. Do the children at least meet these recommendations? Do the parents do so? Some studies suggest that the estimates for time spent in vigorous to moderately vigorous activity in young children should actually be more than this (Hoos *et al.* 2004).

Interpreting the questionnaires

Understanding the relative energy costs of PA (and thus the relative value for weight control) is not easy. One way of comparing the energy expenditure of an activity is through its reported metabolic equivalent or MET (Warburton

Table 10.1. Some methods of assessing physical activity in individuals

Method	Purpose	Description	'Pros' and 'cons'
Prospective assessments			
Step counters	Provide running totals of steps taken within a time period	Small; worn on waist	Relatively objective Fairly cheap Provide immediate feedback to wearer Can be reset and also altered
Pedometers	Can be programmed for stride length as well as step count	Small; worn on waist	As above, but can be used to estimate distance travelled as well as steps taken High accuracy and reliability
Unidimensional accelerometers	Measure movement of limbs and trunk by recording acceleration in up-and-down plane	As above	Similar to the above but more expensive Can be calibrated for energy expenditure and can provide a downloadable record of PA
Tridimensional accelerometers	As above but record movement in three planes Can be programmed for height, weight, age and sex	As above	As above although offering more detail and more expensive
Heart rate monitors	Record intensity of PA by number of heartbeats per minute Heart rate is assumed to relate linearly to oxygen uptake/aerobic fitness	Small; worn around chest with a watch on the wrist Some recent models are worn on the wrist only	Influenced by many factors as well as PA: adrenaline responses, body composition, and temperature Provides a relative profile of PA since there is delay between activity and heart rate change

Table 10.1. (*cont.*)

Method	Purpose	Description	'Pros' and 'cons'
Retrospective assessments			
24-hour recall	Provides a snapshot of activity over the preceding 24 hours	Questionnaire	Clinically useful Convenient to administer Cheap Cost effective Unobtrusive Subject to limitations of memory and the social desirability of responses
Questionnaire of usual activity over a defined period of time	Provides a history of usual and expected activity Informative since activities vary over the course of a week or with time of year and this can be missed in 24-hour recall	Questionnaire	Clinically useful Can recall events with associated timing and intensity Dependent on accuracy of subjective recall Useful adjunct to 24-hour recall

Table 10.2. Minimum physical activity recommended for UK adults and children

	Time	Intensity	Frequency	Current UK situation
Adults	30 minutes	Moderate activity (e.g. brisk walking)	At least 5 days/week	67% men and 75% women do NOT attain this
Children	60 minutes	Moderate activity	Daily	20% boys and 60% girls (2–15 years) do NOT attain this

Source: Chief Medical Officer Report (2004).

et al. 2006b). A MET is the ratio of the metabolic rate of an individual performing a particular task to the resting metabolic rate (RMR) of an average individual. Metabolic equivalents are usually estimated for activity in adults. The oxygen consumption and energy expenditure will not be the same for children as for adults but the proportional effect of the task on the resting metabolism is much the same for many activities (Harrell *et al.* 2005). Some activities will probably have higher MET value for adults and adolescents than for smaller children because larger size (of hands for example) and greater muscular strength enable them to achieve and thus undertake activities that small children can barely manage. Table 10.3 indicates estimated METs for some common activities (Ainsworth *et al.* 2000). Consideration of the MET value of an exercise can be helpful in interpreting activity diaries and responses to questions about daily exercise provided the time spent in an activity is included in any assessment. Vigorous activity uses more energy than moderate or light activity over the same period of time. However an individual may report a vigorous activity lasting a particular period of time but this time includes periods of rest, pauses to get breath back or, in team sports, waiting to have contact with the ball. Periods of less vigorous activity intermingle. Promoting moderate activity with some episodes of vigorous activity may be the most sustainable way of increasing PA especially in relatively unfit overweight/obese children. Walking at MET 2–5 can be maintained by many children and adults for an hour or more. Few are likely to maintain METs of 12.5, even on stationary bicycles at home, for long without pause. Whatever the MET needed for the activity, children are more likely to expend energy if the process of doing so is enjoyable and interesting!

Typically, when asked, individuals report more, or more vigorous, PA than they actually practise. With the overweight/obese, the intensity of any PA tends to be exaggerated because the need to move a bigger body requires more effort and more energy than for the non-obese. Recommendations for time and effort needed for PA in the obese can be made but they should be made on changing what the individual is doing so far rather than on specific

Table 10.3. Metabolic equivalents (METs) for some common activities of childhood

Activity	MET
Moderately vigorous walking	2.5–4.0
Playing guitar	2.0
Making bed	2.0
Dressing	2.0
Walking the dog	3.0
Home play; moderately active with very active periods	4.0
Weeding garden	4.5
Playing games	5.0
Ice skating	5.5
Dancing	6.5
Light to moderately vigorous biking	6.0–8.0
Roller skating	7.0
Jogging	7.0
Playing informal soccer	7.0
Gentle running	8.0
Running upstairs	15.0

Source: Ainsworth *et al.* (2000).

estimations of energy expenditure needed. Overweight/obesity, whatever the present levels of activity, requires more PA than at present to bring weight gain under control.

A few specific questions can give an overview of children's daily activity:

- How do they get to and from school?
- What do they usually do during school breaks?
- How often do they do PE at school?
- Do they enjoy PE at school?
- Do they get hot and sweaty at the end of games and gym? (If not, this suggests they are not putting much effort into the activity.)
- Do they belong to any clubs/classes/activities out of school?
- What do they do at home after school and at weekends?
- Do they play any games/sports outside out of school hours or go cycling with friends, siblings or other relatives?

The benefit of a PA questionnaire is that it describes the activities normally undertaken. It is thus easy to discuss specific activities with children and their families and help them choose where changes might take place to increase energy expenditure and fat loss. Most other methods of recording energy expenditure require some form of activity diary to indicate when and how activity took place.

Table 10.4. Some indicators of relative activity for adults

Overall activity	Steps/day	
Sedentary	<5000	
Low levels of activity	5000–7499	
Moderate levels of activity	7500–9999	
Active	>10 000	

For individual exertion	Breathing	Body temperature
Very light effort	Normal	Normal
Light effort	Slight increase	Start to feel warm
Moderate effort	Greater increase	Warm
Vigorous to very vigorous effort	Difficulty talking and pursuing activity to out of breath and unable to talk	Significantly warm to hot and perspiring heavily

Source: Warbuton *et al.* (2006b).

Motion sensors

Step counters and pedometers are simple, relatively cheap motion sensors available in many sports shops and pharmacies. They provide a summation of body movements with reasonable accuracy (Table 10.1) but give no indication of how that summation is achieved (Warburton *et al.* 2006b). Pedometers can be programmed for stride length as well as number of steps and so provide data on distance covered but they do not record the movement of very slow walking or cycling activity accurately and cannot record water-based activities. From the point of view of managing overweight/obesity they have the big advantage of providing a simple way of setting and monitoring targets for increased PA. Since they are used by competitive walkers and runners when training, pedometers can seem prestigious items rather than something which highlights the problems of the self-conscious overweight.

There are no data on the number of steps taken by children at different ages which equate with specified levels of activity. It may be that, with smaller strides, the number of steps for particular activity levels are similar for adults and children. In Table 10.4 we outline some of the features including step rate which can be used as indicators of levels of activity and of individual activities in adults (Warburton *et al.* 2006b). The proportional increase in steps per day and the physiological effects of individual activities may be similar for children.

What hinders activity in the overweight/obese?

It is easy to tell obese children and their families that they should exercise more. It is easy to tell the children that they should not shirk PE at school or

Table 10.5. Some reasons why obese children may have difficulty increasing formal physical activity

Performing in a very public arena (PE lessons) knowing tasks are executed in a less than flattering manner

Discount PE and express lack of interest in sport and competitive activity to preserve self-esteem

Embarrassment at excessive fat, particularly when changing into more revealing sports gear

Embarrassment due to going red and puffing on exertion

Physical discomfort from folds of fat around thighs chafing with clothing

Orthopaedic problems such as genu valgum causing some difficulty when running

Poor fitness due to low level of physical activity with poor skills and difficulty 'keeping up'

High energy expenditure of moving a heavy body weight compared with a normal body

Rejection by schoolmates and friends as a useful participant in competitive sport

Possible derogatory remarks from PE teachers commenting on performance

that the environment is not so very dangerous and they should walk more or go and play in the park. It is less easy to acknowledge how difficult it can be for overweight and obese children to change their behaviours and to initiate more activity. Parents excuse themselves from activity on the basis of lack of time, lack of finances for gyms and clubs or a dislike of PE instilled at school. These excuses may cover a myriad of other reasons perhaps dating from their own childhoods and can be used to account for why they do not exercise with their children. The children may make similar excuses to cover a number of physical and emotional barriers to participation in PA. If the barriers include bullying and teasing these need addressing.

Table 10.5 lists some of the barriers which come between many overweight/ obese children and enjoyable participation in PA. The actual process of preparing for sports activities at school or at clubs can be misery for these children. They have to change in front of their class, wear the same PE kit and carry out the same tasks. Name-calling and teasing often start as a result of changing for PE lessons. The initial misery may then be exacerbated by not being picked for teams or partnerships or coming last in competitive efforts (Fox and Edmunds 2000). In primary school, some overweight children prefer to participate in formal PA out of school where they are not viewed by their peers. When parents take their overweight children to clubs and classes to encourage activity and energy expenditure their efforts may be thwarted by teachers and coaches who reject the overweight children, not wanting club teams made less competitive or dance classes made less attractive by the presence of the weight encumbered. Too often, by the time overweight children reach secondary school, humiliating episodes such as these have caused them to give up trying to compensate at home for lack of activity in school (Mackett *et al.* 2003; Edmunds and Waters 2004).

How do we increase energy expenditure in physical activity?

Not all obese or overweight children are inactive or lacking sporting prowess. Some, particularly the younger primary school overweight children, are enthusiastic and successful in games and sports. Taller stature and greater weight than many of their peers help in some activities. Thus suggesting to parents that their overweight/obese children are inactive or, even worse, lazy may not be appropriate. Some parents, particularly if they are overweight and not very active themselves, view their children as 'very active' even when other observers draw very different conclusions. Recommendations to increase activity should be accompanied by explanations that however active the children are, increased PA – of almost any variety – should be helpful in controlling weight.

In our experience overweight/obese children rarely show much change in levels of PA until their BMI has fallen a little (after dietary changes). Then, slightly less overweight, the children may be more confident in their ability to achieve, as well as marginally fitter, so they adopt more active lifestyles. Thus attempting to increase overweight children's PA by making small changes in home-based activity initially, coupled with dietary changes which contribute to controlling weight, may be the subtle way to increase fitness and decrease fatness. Once overweight children have become more active, PA can be built up gradually as the children gain in confidence. It may take time for these children to be comfortable with team sports but activities such as dancing, skipping, skating, martial arts and informal activities such as walking and cycling remain useful ways of boosting energy expenditure without involving competition.

Reduce sedentary behaviour

Children seem to follow patterns of being relatively active or relatively sedentary. The motivation for being sedentary is not the same as that for not wanting to be active. Being sedentary may be associated with parental education and family socioeconomic circumstances as well as with the hours spent watching television (Hesketh *et al.* 2006; Janssen *et al.* 2006). Biddle *et al.* (2004) found no significant relationship between physical activity and television viewing. An hour spent in vigorous sport could, in theory at least, be followed by being sedentary for 23 hours. Thus any recommendations for increasing energy expenditure in PA must also make specific recommendations about sedentary behaviours.

We have discussed the role of television in promoting sedentariness in Chapter 8. Advice on weight control must include recommendations about television viewing but children are sedentary not only with television or computers. Many adolescents spend long periods lounging around talking with friends and expending little energy. They are obliged to be sedentary, although intellectually active, when doing homework. Finding ways in which adolescents can be more active within their chosen lifestyles can be difficult and the choices need to come from the adolescents. By contrast parents need to make PA opportunities available to young children. Infants should be placed prone on rugs on floors when they have developed head control, for example, and encouraged to weight bear and then later walk and run around home and garden. It is to be expected that preschool children will exhaust their parents with their activity. Parents may have to channel disorganized restlessness in young children but should try to tolerate normal 'high spirits'. A problem for schools is whether some 'fidgeting' should be more acceptable since it may be one way to help weight control in our children! The difference between sitting absolutely still and wriggling around may be little in terms of METs but the difference accumulated over several hours and days may ultimately have some significance.

Time spent being sedentary can be reduced within the home by encouraging children to take more part in household activities. Throwing the duvet over the bed, tidying the bedroom, loading the dishwasher, helping with gardening, all increase metabolic rates slightly and, if similar light activities take place throughout the day preferably with episodes of moderate to vigorous activity as well, total energy expenditures should increase. The children should benefit socially from being contributing members of the household and from learning simple skills. Many mothers now work full-time as well as running a home. Spending time teaching children simple personal tasks may be seen as time which could be spent doing other things since the mothers could probably do the jobs quicker. However, once children become proficient in such tasks, they relieve their mothers and keep themselves busy. Thus, for example, children should be encouraged to dress themselves from the time when they make their first attempts. Initially they will need a lot of help and some rearrangement of clothing but they need to have mastered dressing by primary school age. Is it relevant that in our clinic many overweight (and sometimes normal weight) children as old as 10 or 11 were helped to undress by their mothers? Does this level of parental help indicate excessive indulgence as a contributing factor to overweight?

Strategies for increasing physical activity

Outside the home small changes in energy expenditure can be made in similar unnoticed ways. Children should be encouraged to walk up stairs rather than use escalators or lifts. Where there are many floors to be climbed perhaps the use of stairs could be graded by going up one floor before taking the lift and then next time going up two floors or getting out a floor early to climb the last stairs. And parents can encourage children to do errands which may be fetching mother's spectacles from upstairs or walking the dog or going to the corner shop (if the shop does not have too many edible temptations).

Walking

Families, and thus children, should walk or cycle wherever possible. Parents should be discouraged from pushing ambulant preschool children in buggies over short distances. Mothers should have some idea of young children's walking limits and encourage them to a walk a little further each time before putting them in the buggy on longish journeys. The use of public transport rather than a car usually involves some walking – maybe only brief – to the bus or railway station.

The journey to school

Walking to school is an opportunity lost for many families. Most primary school children live within 10 minutes of their schools and schools are being encouraged to set up 'walking buses' to take children to school. (In walking buses, responsible adults walk with groups of children from their homes or from collection points to school.) However short the distance from home to school, it seems that if school lies on the route of a parent's car journey to work, the child will be driven to school. Too often mothers drop their children off at school on the way to work because they feel they do not have time to accompany them walking to school and then to go home and drive themselves to work.

Does walking to school really make a difference? In one study from Southern England walking to school did not seem to benefit the total weekly energy expenditure of 5-year-old children significantly (Metcalf et al. 2004). Those who did not walk to school appeared to make up for this lack of exercise by other activities after school or at weekends. However the mean time taken to walk to school in this study was only 6 minutes suggesting that the energy expended in the school journey by these children would have amounted to a very small portion of the weekly total. Another study which used accelerometers to assess activity found primary schoolboys who went to school on foot or by bicycle tended to be more active overall than those who were driven to school (Cooper et al. 2005). Rosenberg et al. (2006) found elementary schoolboys who were active commuters to school had significantly lower average BMI for age than the non-active commuters. Do slimmer boys choose active travel more readily than overweight peers or is the active journey contributing significantly to the control of body fat? Walking to school should do no harm in terms of physical exertion and should have some benefits for cardiorespiratory fitness and energy expenditure in those overweight/obese who otherwise walk very little.

Vigorous activity

The items we have discussed so far mostly involve mild to moderate activity. Episodes of vigorous activity in addition to sustainable increases in moderate PA help promote weight control. Many children need no encouragement to display bouts of very vigorous spontaneous activity. This may result in reprimand for being boisterous in the house or for noisy excited play in the garden – sometimes a very understandable adult response but not helpful to children who need to use up the excess energy stored as fat. Skipping is one activity which can be very brisk and can take place in a small area fairly quietly. Most other very vigorous activity involves running, jumping, throwing or swimming.

Most recommendations for activity as a means of helping reduce overweight/obesity suggest that sustained moderate levels of activity with occasional vigorous activity in addition are effective. Hoos *et al.* (2004) used triaxial accelerometers in young children and found that raising the physical activity level (PAL) significantly – something deemed necessary to have an effect on energy balance – required high-intensity activity. They suggested that the long periods of time young children spend in bed and asleep mean that they need to cram their energy expenditure into a shorter period of time – so the activity has to be more vigorous. Where can young children practise vigorous activity today? Should they be running to school? (Mind the traffic!)

With more mothers working, expecting parents to take children to play in parks or for walks after school is unrealistic for many. Weekends offer time for parents and children to pursue activities to compensate for a lack of activity at other times. This may take some organization and effort on the part of the parents, but this may be the only time some children have to be active, particularly in the winter. Even walking round the shops is preferable in terms of energy expenditure to watching television (although perhaps not preferable in any other way). Being active helps children sleep although vigorous activity and excitement just before bedtime, particularly on light summer evenings, may not be conducive to sleep. Vigorous activity can be followed by a quietening bedtime story.

Implementing change in physical activity

Parents as role models

Significant change in young children's PA is likely to involve parents either by being more active themselves or supporting their children's activity or both.

Since obesity is so frequently familial, this may have health advantages for more members of the family than just the affected children.

Children learn their behaviours from their parents and parents need to be aware of their influence as role models. Parents, particularly of pre-adolescent children, effectively show their children how to be active (or not) as well as supporting the clubs and classes children attend. As Table 10.2 shows, most adults in the UK are not sufficiently physically active so increasing PA as a family can benefit parental health as well as provide the potential enjoyment of family-based outings or social interaction at gyms and sports clubs. Parents who are active participants in sports as adults are more likely to have children who are 'sporty' and have above average levels of fitness (Cleland *et al.* 2005). It is very difficult, even impossible, to motivate children to be more active if the significant adults around them do not value PA and demonstrate their lack of interest or appreciation by continuing to be sedentary.

Walking is an ideal form of exercise for both parents and children. It is habitual, low impact and encourages stamina. Parents can promote their own PA in walking (or other forms of activity) by:

- Setting goals and monitoring progress towards the goals. Write down goals and place the information where all the family can see.
- Finding friendly companions with whom to walk (neighbour, or via organized walks based at the primary care health, or local sports, centres). iPod music and talking books can be helpful distractions for lone walkers.
- Joining a gym or sports club.
- Training for an event with a challenge such as a charity walk.
- Buying a session with a qualified personal trainer to devise an individual walking programme and monitor subsequent progress with log book or pedometer/step counter.
- Changing routes to stop boredom from setting in.
- Having a 'reward' (not edible) when goals are met.

Incremental change in physical activity

The above recommendations can be applied to children as well as adults. A possible programme for increased walking activity for a child might be as follows:

- Make some estimate of steps taken, mileage walked, time spent walking or some other fairly objective assessment of walking activity for one day or one week.
- Set a target of increasing activity by 500 more steps each day for one week and then another 500 steps a day for the next week and so on. Or increase the distance walked/the time spent walking by a specified amount each day for one week and setting a target of walking significantly further the following week.
- Keep an activity logbook to ensure that targets are not being forgotten or ignored.

Change for those who are reluctant to be active with others

Some obese are isolated from friends and reluctant to go out of doors particularly by themselves. They may refuse to engage with a walking programme. When children seem inactive because of lack of friends:

- Find some activity they like doing and increase time spent in this activity.
- Give them pedometers to present them with exercise challenges.
- Choose walks in safe unthreatening environments and challenge them to improve their previous day's PA records.
- Encourage them to dance to music or march on the spot in front of the television.
- Encourage them to work with exercise, dance, yoga, t'ai chi or other PA DVDs/videos at home.
- Take them swimming (even if this is only on holiday).

Any physical activity regime needs to be negotiated with the children/ adolescents in an age-appropriate manner. Activities should be built up in stages so as not to put unfit children off at the beginning of an activity programme. However, putting the onus on children to organize and sustain physical activity regimes by themselves is a little unfair and is likely to fail in the long term. When the children seem ready, they should be encouraged to join in more communal PA. This should provide social support and make PA more likely to be sustained over time.

Introducing a new pattern of behaviour(s) is very difficult, particularly in the early stages. Parents trying to establish a new activity for their child (ideally with family participation) will benefit from the following considerations:

- Plan a regular time for activity:
  Club or class where parents are supportive either financially or through travel arrangements or both
  Sunday walks
- Encourage different members of the family to choose the activities. Activities must be adapted to suit the children whose needs are greatest.
- Identify activities that can engender feelings of achievement and success.
- Allow/encourage indoor play including dancing. Identify suitable areas (garden or beyond) for outdoor activities.
- Play active games with children.
- Select toys which encourage physical activity rather than sedentary behaviours (doll's prams or carts for young children to push; scooters, cycles, pedometers or step counters for those slightly older).
- Reduce time spent watching television, videos, DVDs or playing computer games. Changing these habits may have to be through progressive incremental changes although finding exciting and interesting alternatives to television may help reduce the need to be entertained by television.

- Avoid television in children's bedrooms if possible.
- Offer favourite activities rather than foods as rewards and treats.
- Make PA fun and not necessarily competitive.
- Include friends and relatives at every opportunity.
- Spend as much time out of doors as possible.
- Encourage opportunities for activity at school. Talk to the class teacher about the children's targets for PA.
- Join, or start, a walking school bus.
- Support school projects where being active is a key element.

Informal physical activities

Activity in school is more than just PE and games. There are opportunities at break times for children to play more actively, weather permitting. The most successful obesity prevention interventions for children offer all children active play times either by supplying equipment or instigating short activity programmes. These are inclusive, but require supervisory staff to be interactive which, given the low levels of physical activity in the adult population, may be a stumbling block. There are other issues to bear in mind. Children are more likely to be active in break times if there are balls and other equipment and play items available to them. If the area in which they play is laid out to encourage games (netball, hopscotch, football) or simply a space left free but perhaps patterned imaginatively to encourage inventive play, children are again more likely to be active in break periods. Similarly children will use school PE facilities in free time if there is good functioning equipment available. However play areas can be dominated by active boys who spread out over the area playing football so that girls and less active boys are relegated to the margins. Football-free days or football-free areas may be necessary since overweight and obese (and some normal weight) children may not be prepared to participate in playground team games as they are likely to feel unacceptable even without having to change clothes. Clubs and classes based on individual activities such as line dancing and t'ai chi may be more acceptable to children but such classes must avoid becoming exercise classes only for the overweight and obese since this is likely to increase the stigma and isolation already inflicted by schoolmates.

When presented appropriately, PA provides children with the opportunity to improve their self-confidence and self-esteem, and gives them a sense of achievement and a sense of inclusion. These social benefits are potentially very important. If children are having fun, they worry less about their appearance. The active overweight may need little encouragement to do more but this may be constrained by practical considerations such as parents' lack of time and finances if supervision outside the home is required. Children who have learned from experience that PA is embarrassing and painful are more difficult to engage in activity. For them, PA comprises a set of behaviours which have been discounted as areas where they lack competence and recognition of this undermines their sense of self-worth. They have to learn that PA can be fun. Their PA needs to be in an acceptable form, initially probably taking place largely out of school and on an individual basis.

If children are adamant they will not take part in school PE or games, parents and teachers should try to find out why this is so. If it is because of embarrassment changing or when dressing in sports outfit, there may be room for some negotiation over school policies for PE particularly as there may be several other children with the same problems. If the delivery, attitude or language of the PE games teacher is having a negative effect, parents should again try to discuss this with the teacher or with the school head-teacher. Ordering or trying to force overweight children to take part in formal activity is unlikely to succeed and will reinforce negative attitudes. It will not convert sport-phobics to sport-philics! It is inevitable that some overweight children cannot be persuaded to take part in PE and for them PE has to be abandoned as an energy expenditure opportunity. Out of school activities must be all the more intense and sustained to make up for lack of PE in school.

Should we buy him/her an exercise bicycle?

This question is often posed by parents of children who have little interest in activity as PE at school or in playing outside with friends. An exercise bicycle seems to offer opportunity for the child to exercise without the opprobrium of jeering friends and neighbours. However home exercise bicycles are not enormously sturdy and often quite uncomfortable for the overweight to ride. Physical problems of fat thighs rubbing together or the reach of the pedals being wrong for the child are combined with the fact that most people find exercise bicycles a very boring way of being active. Children could ride on the bicycle in the living room whilst watching television but cycling may diminish as the television becomes more engrossing. Other members of the family may complain that their view of the television is blocked by the apparatus. To be useful exercise, a child should probably cycle sufficiently vigorously to feel very warm for a period of half an hour a day minimum.

Exercise bicycles are too frequently permanent residents of junk room or garage – lost to use. Families would be wise to see if they can borrow one of these pieces of apparatus, or at least give the child a chance to try a cycle out thoroughly, before they spend significant amounts of money on a piece of apparatus which may be quickly rejected by the child as too difficult, too uncomfortable or too boring.

Swimming

Swimming, as well as being an important skill for all children to acquire, is the best and worst activity for the obese. The overweight are often good swimmers, being buoyant, strong and with stamina. However the ordeal of changing and walking to the pool with their figure exposed may cause these children to give up swimming. Assuming their parents do not have their own pool, children should use holiday times as good opportunities to practise swimming. On holiday, the overweight do not have to face their classmates or the school bullies whilst in their bathing costumes. They can enjoy themselves.

The rewards

Overweight/obese children should be praised for taking part in PA and for their achievements in PA even though their achievements may seem less impressive than those of their normal weight peers. A positive supportive approach, which is not patronizing, encourages children to pursue activities further – something which applies to all children irrespective of their body status.

Table 10.6. Summary of approaches to implementing greater physical activity

Reduce time spent sitting and relaxed
Reduce television viewing
Develop a helpful busy attitude towards other members of household
Encourage errands for family members which require going up and down stairs
Encourage personal care and independence: dressing, tidying bedroom, making bed
Increase time spent moving about rapidly: in the home, outside the house, at school
Increase time spent in informal active play both at home and in school breaks
Increase time spent in:
    school sports
    gym
    formal and informal ball games
    dancing, skipping, singing games
    cycling, walking
    skating, swimming, martial arts

Recommendations

- Increasing PA and making PA enjoyable should be essential to all programmes of weight control for overweight/obese children.
- Physical activity is many-faceted. Physical activity can be increased across a range of life skills (Table 10.6).
- In developing individual programmes to increase PA parents must be involved and even encouraged to increase their own PA.
- Documenting daily activity can challenge overweight children to achieve more each day. Documentation may be through activity diaries, time spent in specific activities or with pedometers or step counters.
- Increased moderate activity, especially activity such as walking which requires nothing innovative, will probably be more sustainable long term than unwelcome attempts to increase children's vigorous activity significantly. However fat loss and lowered BMI, perhaps as a result of dietary change, may result in beneficial but spontaneous increases in vigorous activity.
- Adolescents should develop their own plans for increased activity. Primary care set-ups may be helpful here if the adolescents feel they will lose face developing activity plans with their parents but, to create the right ambience, primary care facilities must have adolescent-friendly features (Royal College of General Practitioners/Royal College of Nursing 2002).
- All programmes to increase PA must include elements which focus on decreasing time spent being sedentary as well as time spent being obviously active.

11

What else can be done?

This book is concerned with first-line approaches to the management of childhood overweight and obesity. Drug treatment and surgical interventions are not first-line management. They are not solutions for those who are non-compliant with diet or other standard management. Interventions with drugs or surgery should only be considered for adolescents and children when their overweight/obesity has been investigated and assessed thoroughly by a paediatric team experienced in managing overweight children. For obese adults, drugs and surgery can contribute to management in some severely affected obese and in those with co-morbidities. Paediatric services are beginning to define young people, adolescents in particular, for whom drug treatment or bariatric surgery may usefully complement other weight management practices. Thus we feel it is important that those treating all over-weight/obese children should have some knowledge of the children who might benefit from pharmaceutical or surgical interventions, particularly since these primary care teams may be involved in the follow up management of these children.

The recent NICE (2006) Guidelines on the management of overweight/obesity do accept that some children and adolescents benefit from drug treatment or from bariatric surgery. However no drug is currently licensed for use in childhood obesity in the UK although licenses for use with adolescents are being sought. Surgery should be confined to children who are at real risk from the complications of their obesity and, because surgery can occasionally lead to nutritional inadequacies, have completed or almost completed growth and physical maturation.

Drugs

The only two drugs currently licensed for treatment of obesity in UK adults, orlistat and sibutramine, are, at the time of writing not licensed for treatment

Table 11.1. Possible use of drugs for treatment of overweight/obese children

Children under 12 years	Children 12 years and over	Both age groups

• Drug treatment not generally recommended
• Drug treatment may be used only in exceptional circumstances, e.g. severe life-threatening co-morbidities:
    sleep apnoea
    raised intracranial
    pressure
	• Drug treatment only recommended if physical co-morbidities present, e.g. orthopaedic problems, sleep apnoea and/or severe psychological co-morbidities	• Drug treatment should be initiated and progress followed by a multidisciplinary team with expertise in:
		    drug monitoring
		    psychological support
		    behavioural
		        interventions
		    interventions to
		        increase activity
		    interventions to
		        improve diet
		• Drugs should only be prescribed if the prescriber is willing to submit data to the proposed national registry on the use of these drugs in young people
		• Once drug treatment has begun it may be continued in primary care if local circumstances and/or licensing allow this

of those under 18 years old. Other drugs are also under study in adults (Padwal and Majumdur 2007). Research studies using these drugs for obesity have been almost exclusively involved with individuals over 18 years of age. NICE (2006) Guidelines make suggestions for the possible use of these drugs with overweight/obese children as shown in Table 11.1.

Orlistat

Orlistat is taken in conjunction with meals and acts by inhibiting a range of intestinal lipases so reducing fat absorption by about 30%. The unabsorbed fat passes through the bowel resulting in fatty stools. Urgency, frequent defaecation and leakage of oily faecal material can be undesirable consequences of treatment but are minimized by a low fat diet. Thus taking the drug usually reduces energy intake as well as energy absorption from the bowel. Apart from causing the unpleasant side effects on bowel function, the drug has the potential to precipitate fat-soluble vitamin malabsorption. A micronutrient supplement providing the recommended daily nutrient intake of all minerals and vitamins is recommended by NICE (2006) for those who may be put at risk of deficiency by malabsorption. Children's growth and nutrition would certainly seem at risk from the drug treatment so micronutrient supplementation should be prescribed. If the drug is used in those under the age of 18, there should be regular monitoring of growth, calcium, phosphate and alkaline phosphatase levels and even bleeding and clotting times since the fat-soluble vitamins are the most likely to become deficient. This need to monitor blood biochemistry regularly may be a negative factor for obese children who are often reluctant to submit to 'investigations'.

NICE (2006) recommends orlistat for use in adults only:

- after dietary, exercise and behavioural approaches have been started and evaluated
- in adults who classify as obese (BMI 30 or more) or who have slightly lower degree of overweight (BMI 28 or more) and associated risk factors
- in those who have not reached their target weight loss or who have reached a plateau in weight loss on diet, exercise and behavioural change
- after its use has been extensively discussed with the patient and the patient has been counselled on additional diet, exercise and behavioural strategies associated with use of the drug
- for more than 3 months if the patient has lost at least 5% of initial body weight in the 3 months from starting treatment. Therapy beyond 12 months should only be considered after extensive discussion with the patient of the benefits and limitations of long-term treatment with the drug. Two years is the maximum duration of treatment recommended.

Sibutramine

Sibutramine affects the level of serotonin in the brain by inhibiting the reuptake of noradrenaline and serotonin in the brain. It seems to act by causing feelings of satiety and thus suppressing appetite. Side effects include increased BP, tachycardia, headaches, dry mouth, constipation and sleep problems. As with orlistat it is not licensed for use in children. It should be avoided in those with hypertension and cardiovascular problems as well as those with significant psychiatric disturbance.

NICE (2006) recommendations for use of sibutramine in adults are similar to those for orlistat in that use is recommended only as part of an overall plan of management in adults who classify as obese (BMI 30 or more) or have slightly lower degree of overweight than for orlistat (27 or more) and have associated risk factors (type 2 diabetes mellitus or dyslipidaemia). It should only be prescribed if there are adequate arrangements for checking for adverse effects such as hypertension. The recommendations for use beyond 3 months' duration are as with orlistat and treatment is usually only recommended for 1 year.

Neither of these two drugs should be used in combination with each other nor with other drugs intended to help weight reduction.

It should be clear from this that drug treatment for overweight/obesity in children is not something that should be instituted lightly and certainly not without significant preceding effort to control weight by other means except when life-threatening conditions make fat loss urgent. In such cases the affected children should be under specialist paediatric supervision anyway.

Metformin

Metformin is a biguanide drug which acts by decreasing gluconeogenesis and increasing peripheral utilization of glucose. Its role is in management of type 2 diabetes mellitus. However it has been shown to be of use in reducing weight (compared with matched controls) and improving insulin sensitivity in non-diabetic adults with obesity and reduced insulin sensitivity (Charles *et al.* 2000). A few small, short, studies in children under 18 with hyperinsulinaemia and obesity but no diabetes have shown greater weight/BMI loss in the group given metformin (Freemark and Bursey 2001; Kay *et al.* 2001; Lustig *et al.* 2006). Whether the drug also had positive metabolic effects was not stated. These studies have led to questions whether metformin has a place in reducing overweight and helping prevent deterioration of insulin sensitivity in obese adolescents and even children. Currently there is no good evidence that this is the case and use of the drug is confined to obese type 2 diabetic children. As with the other drugs discussed here, its use should be instigated only by those experienced in managing children with obesity, reduced insulin sensitivity and type 2 diabetes who are working in tertiary level paediatric centres.

Bariatric surgery

Surgical treatment of obesity is now a widely accepted management for selected severely obese adults but it is not generally recommended as management for individuals under 18 years. Nevertheless it has been used in younger people from time to time – usually in adolescents and sometimes as a rather desperate measure when other efforts to control severe obesity have failed. Families may request surgical treatment for their obese children or

HCPs may wonder whether particular adolescents or children under their care would benefit from surgery. It is important therefore to understand the circumstances in which children may benefit from surgical procedures for their obesity. Whilst usually seen as an adjunct to diet and exercise in the morbidly obese adolescent, there is a view that surgery should not be seen as 'last ditch' management but as a more or less routine procedure in the very severely obese so as to protect them from the physical and psychological disadvantages likely to affect them in adult life (Garcia and De Maria 2006; Inge *et al.* 2007). We therefore outline possible indications for surgery and some surgical procedures here.

NICE (2006) Guidelines recommend considering bariatric surgery for children only in exceptional circumstances. Children should be more or less fully grown and physiologically mature. Surgery should be undertaken only if there are facilities for:

- pre-operative assessment including thorough medical examination with screening for genetic causes for obesity, specialist assessment for eating disorders and risk–benefit analysis incorporating consideration of the prevention of complications of obesity
- providing information on the various procedures including plastic surgery such as apronectomy, on the relative risks of surgery and on the likely effect of surgery for overweight versus the possible risks if surgery is not undertaken
- regular post-operative assessment with specialist surgical and dietetic follow-up
- management of co-morbidities
- psychological support both before and after surgery
- follow-up by staff trained in the procedures and in the rehabilitation of post-operative obese children
- comprehensive psychological, educational, family and social assessments before children are accepted for surgery
- surgical care and follow up which is in accordance with Children's National Service Framework core standards.

This seems a long list but many items should be routinely provided by a specialist surgical team managing childhood obesity. It is very important that the last recommendation is implemented. The ambience of the surgical ward must be appropriate for obese children. Staff should be not only trained in managing bariatric surgery cases but also experienced with nursing adolescents and children. Children need to be in children's wards or children's hospitals. Adolescents are not appropriately managed on wards full of infants and toddlers but are equally 'out of water' in surgical wards occupied by overweight middle-aged men and women, for example. Thus selection of the unit for surgical management of childhood obesity is very important. Needless to say, surgeons must be experienced not only in bariatric surgical procedures but also appropriately trained in operating on the young obese. There is a long list of possible complications of bariatric surgery (Speiser *et al.* 2005) although obese children are probably no more prone to these than are obese adults.

What operations are done?

Although intestinal bypass operations are still sometimes performed, many bariatric surgical procedures nowadays are varieties of gastric banding (Kral 2006). Gastric banding is a fairly simple procedure which can be carried out laparoscopically and is potentially reversible (Yitzhak *et al.* 2006). A silastic band placed around the cardia of the stomach creates a small upper stomach pouch. The silastic band can be adjusted through a small subcutaneous port thus changing the size of the exit from the pouch and the readiness with which the subject feels 'full'. The small upper pouch tends to prohibit eating a lot of food at any one time thus reducing energy intake although frequent high energy liquid meals can counter the effects of surgery in non-compliant subjects.

With the development of more sophisticated methods of gastric banding, bypass operations have become less common, particularly with young people. The bypass operations commonly practised are Roux en Y procedures (Lawson *et al.* 2006) where a small gastric pouch is created by stapling off part of the cardia of the stomach and linking a section of the jejunum with the pouch. The duodenum is effectively bypassed creating some malabsorption as well as easy satiety from stomach restriction. If the malabsorption creates significant micronutrient malabsorption this could damage growth in children who are not fully mature. Bypass operations are more complicated than gastric banding, although they too can be done laparoscopically. They are not easy to reverse. More drastic procedures such as the removal of a portion of the stomach and linking a section of the jejunum with the gastric pouch seem less desirable as procedures for children.

Complications

The immediate risks of any form of surgery in obese children are greater, as with adults, than in normal weight children. Thus it is important to have a team skilled in paediatric surgery as well as bariatric techniques and in managing obese children. The ability to perform bariatric surgery via laparoscopic approaches reduces the risks of abdominal surgery but the risks need to be balanced against potential benefits.

In the long term the operations are not entirely free of problems. Gastric banding reduces the size of the stomach pouch. Discomfort and/or vomiting may be associated with inadequate chewing of food, eating too rapidly so the pouch overfills, or even drinking soon after eating. If there is persistent vomiting the gastric pouch may stretch thus reducing the beneficial effect of the small 'stomach'. Initial follow-up may require fairly frequent attendances to adjust the gastric band so pouch size is appropriate for reasonable weight loss in each child. With time the stomach pouch increases in size and the effect on weight reduction may be reduced. With operations where there is an enterostomy and some bowel is bypassed there is need for long-term regular follow-up – perhaps annually – after the initial year but more frequent early follow-up as there is the potential for malabsorption of micronutrients. Micronutrient status needs checking biochemically at least annually (Kral 2006).

Adolescents and children who have had gastric banding or some other operation in which stomach size is reduced need to be advised to eat carefully. They should eat slowly, making sure they chew their food well. They should drink before eating or leave drinks until more than an hour after food. If they feel full they should stop eating. If they vomit they should avoid food and drink for 4 hours and then try drinking before eating again. If vomiting persists they should seek medical advice.

Initial weight losses are impressive with surgery but weight loss often flattens out so that by 2 years after surgery, differences in BMI loss between those receiving the most and those receiving the least radical procedures are almost undetectable. In adults, mortality from obesity co-morbidities is less in those who have had bariatric surgery than those of equivalent BMI managed by non-invasive management (Kral 2006).

Prader–Willi syndrome and surgery

Surgical procedures have been used in PWS despite the difficulties of ensuring an affected child is fully conversant with the implications of the operation. For many of these children and their parents surgery can provide respite from the rigid dietary processes necessary to keep weight under control. However, if these children have undisciplined eating, bariatric surgery may do little good and might even be dangerous. The parents must feel that their child's eating can be restrained so they eat slowly, chew and can be prevented from eating excessively. Without these provisos, maintaining smaller well-masticated meals may be impossible and vomiting, operative failure or other difficulties may ensue. Thus, whether or not to suggest a PWS child has surgery is a difficult decision. The risks from surgery are above average and the benefits from surgery potentially lower than for 'normal' overweight children because PWS children may not contain their eating even though their gastric band does limit intake over any one short period.

Recommendations

- Drugs and bariatric surgery added to other actions to control weight can be effective in children whose obesity has failed to respond well to other measures.
- These treatments are not without risk and should only be undertaken after broad assessment of the affected children and after extensive discussion with the child and its family.
- These are managements for those trying to control their obesity and are not for those who are not prepared to make efforts to deal with their weight problems – or those of their children.
- NICE Guidelines give quite clear instructions for the use of drugs and surgery in children and adolescents and these should be followed at the present time.
- In the future these lines of management may become more routine practice. We should prefer a reduction in the prevalence of childhood obesity so that there is also a reduction in the need for these therapies.

12

How can we sustain healthy weight management?

One of the problems for those obese and overweight who manage to control their weight successfully is preventing the gradual (or rapid) return to previous overweight. As children grow up and develop physiologically and psychologically, lifestyle changes may become embedded with the consequences that weight status may be easier to maintain than for adults adapting to modifications of already entrenched lifestyles. Many obese and overweight children do continue as obese and overweight adults but the correlation between obesity in childhood and in adult life is greatest when the time between the two assessments is short. As a generalization, the younger the child or the further from childhood the adult is, the lower the correlation between overweight/obesity in childhood and in adult life. As childhood and adult overweight and obesity become increasingly common, the chances of an overweight or obese child remaining overweight or obese as an adult will increase since overweight adults are unlikely to come equally from children of all weight states. Even so, the majority of obese adults were normal weight children and a significant proportion of overweight children do slim down either before the end of childhood or in adult life.

If we are to build on change which may occur naturally anyway, the processes of achieving sustainable normal BMI or significant loss of fat require considerable time. Children and families seeking help for weight problems usually have initial enthusiasm to act but rarely recognize how slow the process of 'slimming' can be. As time passes the enthusiasm and effort put into weight control can wane. Unless the family and child have by then adopted significant differences to their lifestyles, the success of the fat reducing process may also wane. What can be done to help maintain weight control and, ideally, progressive lowering of BMI until the normal range of BMI is reached?

We have discussed the importance of retaining a positive approach to the child and family in relation to weight control. We have also discussed providing a clinic or weight group environment which is friendly and helpful and enjoyable for children and their families. What are also needed are clubs and youth groups where the overweight child can go with confidence to meet with peers and be active and social following enjoyable healthy pursuits. Time, growth, greater independence and maturity give children and adolescents greater control over their own lives. Eventually leaving home leads to what are often significant differences in lifestyles and degrees of overweight. Sadly if the next home is a university hall or a house where students cater for themselves on low budgets, diets may deteriorate in quality. The solution to weight control then lies in maintaining high levels of activity. These are changes that occur because of the development of the children within and without the family. What else can be done to give support to the weight controlling process?

Reinforcement

Most successful weight control programmes for children are associated with frequent contacts between HCPs and overweight children and their families. We recommend that children with weight problems are reviewed 2 weeks after their first visit and every 2 to 4 weeks after that until they and their families feel confident that they can make progress with less frequent attendances. However attendances cannot be imposed. Families must be given choice about the frequency of attendance since, particularly if the clinic or weight control group is distant from home, they may be keen for reasons of time and finance to spread out appointments. If the demands for attendances are too great, attendances will lapse. For older children, missing school if an attendance is during school hours can be a problem partly because it draws the attention of their schoolmates to the overweight but also because schoolwork becomes increasingly important as children move up their schools. A compromise between what might be most desirable for maintaining action on weight control needs to be balanced against the child and family's perceptions of what is practical for them. Timing clinics for evenings or Saturday mornings to suit adolescent children and their working parents may help enthusiastic follow-up but also requires above-average enthusiasm from the HCP.

What should be done when children attend for follow-up?

When children and families re-attend the clinic or advice centre, the HCP wants to know how well they have succeeded in implementing the lifestyle changes they chose and in following the advice previously given. Parents and children may give rather different stories about their success with weight control. Sometimes both parents and children give very optimistic views of their efforts and dramatic descriptions of how weights have changed on the bathroom scales. Whilst all effort should be encouraged, it is wise to avoid vigorous congratulation until the children have been weighed and measured in the clinic and BMI calculated. Weight gain since the previous attendance can create doubt about the value of families' description of action taken. The HCP will need to work discreetly around the topic of what changes have really been achieved at home. What are the problems – the barriers (Murtagh *et al.* 2006)?

Discussion centres on what the child has attempted in relation to targets suggested at the previous attendance. What have been the difficulties and problems encountered? Has the child become spontaneously more active? Is the child more self-confident and showing evidence of more positive social interaction (if this was a problem previously)? What are the difficulties for other family members involved in the weight controlling process?

Children are weighed and their heights measured preferably in only light underclothes although undressing to this extent may not be acceptable to all. Shoes must be removed. BMI is calculated and weight, height and BMI are plotted on growth charts. The data will indicate one of the following:

- BMI has fallen (with loss of weight, no change in weight or even small increment if height has increased)
- there has been no noticeable change in weight or BMI
- there has been a significant increase in BMI and an increase in weight.

The child who has lost weight or reduced BMI should be congratulated but with the clear proviso that this is only the beginning of the weight controlling process. There may be a need to 'plateau' for a while at the current level of change – particularly if it is proving effective in controlling weight gain. Or a new round of targets for incremental change can be discussed with child and parents and a subsequent appointment arranged. It is important for the family to realize that they have achieved something and can congratulate themselves *but* that they should continue vigilance of the child's lifestyle and continue weight control efforts. Too often initial success is seen as something which the family should celebrate with the child. They go to a café and reward the child with edible treats – and the efforts put into changing habits and tastes and controlling energy intake over the previous weeks are wasted.

If there is no significant change in BMI, although perhaps a little disappointing, the family should be encouraged to recognize that (after the first years) normal BMI rises with age so maintenance of BMI is in itself an achievement. An appointment after only 2 weeks' efforts can mean that there has been insufficient time for change to be measurable. This can be particularly true for adolescent girls where weight may vary throughout the monthly cycle with water retention – and some increase in weight – towards the end of the menstrual cycle. Careful discussion may reveal areas of action where efforts to make changes have slipped and unimpressive progress can be explained. If nothing is revealed to explain slow progress, the family should be encouraged that as they build up lifestyle changes greater weight change is likely.

Families where there has been no progress in even controlling rate of weight gain are the most difficult to handle. The picture of diet and activity described by the child may sound ideal although the weight indicates that circumstances are likely to be otherwise. The family's description of efforts made may be entirely genuine even though evidence of immediate success has eluded them. It may be appropriate to explain that the propensity for obesity is stronger in some children than others and it may be that this child will only show weight change with increased dietary and exercise interventions. If the attendance is early in the period of management, it may be that longer is needed before small incremental changes begin to have sufficient effect to be recorded on clinic scales. Additional targets for change in diet and activity are set and another appointment arranged in the near future. Sometimes where it is doubtful whether the family really are making the efforts described it may be necessary to point out it is what happens outside the clinic, not what is described in the clinic, that effects change.

Some non-responders continue to attend for weight control advice without ever seeming to put into effect the changes they choose or the advice they are given. Certainly there are no reductions in their overweight or obesity. This may be because the children/adolescents are avoiding all attempts to change their lifestyles and, not surprisingly, BMI is not improving. Failure of children to cooperate with parents' attempts to help their weight problem can result in increasing tension and friction between parents and affected children. Is the result worth the confrontation? At some stage advisor, family and child need to come to an agreement that attendance at the clinic is not, per se, slimming. Persistent failure to make any progress is wasting child and family's time as well as that of their advisor. The child should be politely dropped from clinic attendance after a repetition of advice on possible lifestyle, diet and activity changes. Discharge from the clinic or weight control group should be on friendly terms if at all possible. Should these still overweight children decide sometime in the future that they wish to pursue active weight reduction, they should feel able to return for advice without shame or embarrassment.

Incremental changes

We have suggested that change should be by small incremental stages. It is important to continue to build on these in ways which are practical for families. As presented in this book it may seem that the changes we recommend should all take place at once. This is generally an impossible undertaking for families and almost certainly unsustainable long term. Families and children need to target changes they think they can achieve initially and then be introduced gradually to more and more significant changes. Building up to the dietary and activity changes we indicate will take time. Families may need to gain confidence in their ability to change behaviours. Separating changes into those primarily for parents to implement and those for the children to implement may lead to several changes taking place as each family member assumes responsibility for something. Thus the child may be prepared to cut out some snacks whilst father might plan to grill foods without added fat on the cooker in the kitchen just as he does on the barbecue. Mother might plan to take the child out at weekends when she goes jogging. When seen next time, perhaps the child might be prepared to cut down sweetened drinks, mother might introduce more energy reduced versions of food brands and family activity could be more vigorous or for longer. A diary of step changes might help all to see the build-up of change and the effects they were having – and feel inspired to look for what to do next.

As the children's BMIs fall closer to normal for age the children often become spontaneously more active. They enjoy being active more and they find it less difficult to be active. Whilst early changes in lifestyles may focus on reducing sedentariness and adopting less energy dense diets and more controlled eating, with time the focus of weight control may turn more to increased PA. However, throughout attendances children and their families should be offered nutritional advice which will help them make future healthy choices over foods, even if a sustainable healthy diet has been established and there is no longer need to make further dietary change. It is difficult for those who know little about nutrition to grasp all that they may be being told at a few attendances. Further, from time to time bizarre nutritional recommendations circulate in the media or in public culture and these may need to be discussed and exposed. Advice needs repeating and concepts must be explained in ways which are comprehensible to the family and where appropriate the children. Children are sometimes the ones who point out to parents where wrong decisions are being made.

Signing off

Many children attending for weight consultations lose some weight and show significant falls in BMI but do not return to totally normal BMI. They may plateau at a level of overweight considerably less than that with which they first attended. How long should they continue to attend? Often the children and family decide that they can continue to manage the child's weight themselves and ask to stop attending. With some families attendance becomes a routine where there is little change and the family is following the best lifestyle they are probably able to achieve. If the situation is stable there will come a time when it is probably appropriate to stop attendances perhaps by first lengthening the period between reviews to 2 to 3 months and then 6 months before suggesting attendance stops. If there are gyms or clubs where the child – or perhaps by now young adult – can go to focus on PA and healthy living this may be a good way to graduate from the weight control group or clinic. Primary care trusts should perhaps consider developing links with such gyms/clubs – if they do not already exist – perhaps through special category membership.

It should always be made clear to discharged children and families that those who find their weight getting out of control again are welcome back for further help and advice.

Recommendations

- First review after weight control advice should be within 2 to 4 weeks from the first visit.
- The overarching aim is for families to change their behaviours to live healthier lifestyles.
- For children, learning sustainable change involves parents encouraging them in appropriate for age autonomy and responsibility so they can gradually become independent of external motivation when effecting lifestyle change.
- Progress and difficulties with diet and activity change should be discussed at each visit.
- Weight, height and BMI of the children should be measured, calculated and recorded at each attendance.
- The weight and BMI findings should be shown to the family and discussed, preferably using weight and BMI for age charts to illustrate the changes since the previous attendance.
- Even small changes should be applauded and lack of change should be treated as perhaps an indication that a little longer is needed before change will show or that there is need for greater lifestyle change.
- The need and desire for further changes should be considered with child and family and new targets set for lifestyle changes
- Further follow-up should be planned but some goal should be developed as progress is made so attendance does not drag on indefinitely.
- It may be helpful for the weight control clinic/group to establish a special relationship with sports clubs and gyms in the area so children can pursue

PA and possibly have their weight kept under review once discharged from the clinic/group set-up.

- Children who control their weight well may be reassured by very infrequent – e.g. annual – reviews once they have achieved sufficient BMI change.
- Groups and clinics dealing with overweight subjects need exit strategies both for non-cooperative attendees and for successful attendees.

13

What can we do to prevent childhood overweight and obesity?

The rapidly rising incidence of overweight/obesity amongst both adults and children in many westernized countries suggests that control of the obesity epidemic will depend on effective programmes to prevent overweight developing rather than on more effective management, important though this latter aspect is. Yet, just as there is no consensus view on the specific details for management of overweight/obesity in childhood, so there is no consensus view on effective prevention. A review of studies, many of which were from North America, on the prevention of overweight/obesity in children found some studies which fulfilled the Cochrane criteria for objective analysis and, of those included in the review, none came out with impressively effective plans for prevention (Summerbell *et al.* 2005). However some interventions were at early stages in their implementation. Many showed some evidence of changes in behaviours (Summerbell *et al.* 2005). Thus there is plenty of opportunity for properly conducted, randomized control studies designed to reduce the prevalence of overweight/obesity in present-day child populations.

Some overweight prevention studies have focused on only one contributor to overweight, for example diet. Sustainable weight control and overweight prevention needs broad changes in lifestyles for most families. Measures to prevent overweight should impact on behaviours around diet and activity but also include the family environment. Intervening to modify only diet or only activity is largely ineffective (Anderson 2002).

Constructing effective preventive programmes is complicated by the wide range of stakeholders who are, or could be, involved in programmes for weight control in childhood. As well as children, these include families, schools, communities, local and national governments, the media, commerce – and others (Figure 13.1). A range of geographical and social differences impact on weight status so that for a particular child, or for children in one community, the immediate risk factors for overweight in home and environment may be very different from those affecting other children and other

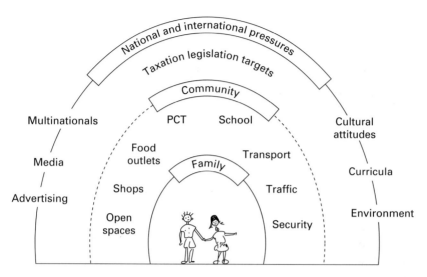

Figure 13.1 Societal pressures on children which influence weight and weight control.

communities. In many cases we do not know which are the specific risk factors for particular groups – but just that some groups have increased risk. For example, we have no easy explanation for the differences in prevalence of overweight/obesity amongst children from different ethnic groups (Whincup et al. 2002; Viner et al. 2006). Genetic endowment may be one factor but environmental issues and family aspirations and expectations are probably more important for most of these children. The scope of preventive interventions needs to be wide in the hope of encompassing all unrecognized contributory factors in change.

Who is at risk?

Prevention can be interpreted as primary prevention which aims to reduce the incidence of a condition; secondary prevention which aims to reduce the prevalence of the condition; and tertiary prevention which aims to reduce the severity and complications of the conditions (World Health Organization 1998). Our aim here is to discuss primary prevention since secondary and tertiary prevention have, in effect, been covered by earlier chapters on the management of childhood overweight and obesity.

The first line of prevention for many medical conditions is defining who is 'at risk' and then developing methods of finding and involving the 'at risk' population. The current prevalence of childhood overweight in most industrialized countries and the predicted increases over the next few years suggest that we should consider the whole childhood population in these countries as at risk of developing overweight. In each population there will be some groups who are at particular risk, for example certain age groups. This may be because changing behaviours as part of development at certain ages make it critical that healthy eating habits and active lifestyles are incorporated into those behavioural changes. Or it may be because the risks of overweight are physiologically greater in one gender, one age, or perhaps one ethnic group within a society. In our view the weaning period and adolescence are the two age groups which deserve special consideration. School entry may be another time when children are vulnerable to new peer-inspired ways of eating and spending leisure time. School policies – and the Healthy Schools Programme – are very important for this age group (Department of Health 2007a). Apart from age related periods of vulnerability we list the particularly vulnerable as:

- those with a family history of overweight
- those with certain specific medical conditions known to be associated with overweight /obesity
- those with physical disability which causes reduced ability to be physically active
- those from deprived environments where understanding of healthy lifestyles, access to healthy foods and access to safe open spaces may be limited
- those with emotional or learning difficulties and/or poor social skills which lead to isolation amongst peers.

Primary prevention – aiming to stop children becoming overweight in the first place – broadly overlaps with management. Most of the suggestions we have made for the management of childhood overweight by changing life-styles to create sustainable weight control can be applied, possibly more successfully, to primary prevention of childhood overweight/obesity. The range of possible preventive actions is enormous and the variety of pro-grammes that have been tried or are being tried likewise immense. We cannot cover all suggested approaches here. Thus, we focus on measures which relate to primary care and the community although touching upon wider issues in relation to the media, advertising and governmental action. For example, many preventive measures such as better-quality school dinners and more activity-friendly environments, which are essentially issues for the commu-nity, are likely to be implemented more readily with financial, legislative and other backing from governments.

If preventive programmes are aimed at whole populations it is important that the programmes should not increase the risk of malnutrition for normal weight individuals in the population. Major emphasis on losing weight, looking slim and reducing energy intake could draw emotionally and psy-chologically vulnerable individuals towards the development of eating disorders: bulimia and anorexia nervosa. Thus programmes dealing with the prevention of overweight should stress positive action such as 'healthy life-styles', sensible eating, the enjoyment of physical activity and sport rather than focus on losing weight, body shape, dieting and 'calories'. Similarly those trying to educate the clinic or community population on the prevention of overweight need to be sensitive to the possible presence of susceptible individuals who will misinterpret advice. Recognizing children in whom there is inappropriate dieting or weight loss when they are not overweight, or recognizing those who seem very concerned about what they eat even though they are already thin, should lead to sensitive inquiry about what is really happening (Pugliese *et al.* 1983). In addition to those schoolchildren and adolescents who diet unnecessarily and sometimes pathologically, there are also some parents who become overconcerned about the possibility of their children becoming obese. They follow healthy diet messages obsessively to the extent that their children, particularly if still preschool, receive inadequate nutrition (Morgan *et al.* 2006). Early dietary restriction too rigidly managed may even predispose to obesogenic eating later (Clark *et al.* 2007).

Prevention at home

Where children's ages make it appropriate, family policies about eating, activity, television viewing, bedtimes and other matters should be discussed and policies developed and agreed with the children (Dixon-Woods *et al.* 1999) (Table 13.1). These may be family-wide agreements but for age dependent matters they will probably be developed separately for each child.

At-risk ages

Weaning

Diet
Developing lifestyles which help reduce the incidence of overweight should begin in early life so they become habitual. However, the first 6 months of life, when children are fully breast fed or entirely formula fed, is not an appropriate time to restrict the energy intake and increasing energy expenditure at that age is neither easy nor practical. If children are fed infant formula and are gaining weight at rates greater than expected from increases in length, it is sensible to check that the formula is made up correctly, that weaning foods are not being offered early, that frequency of feeds is reasonable and that the children are not being satiated with bottles when they are really hungry for the company and stimulation of their carers. Some rapid

Table 13.1. Recommendations for prevention at the family level

Diet	Activity	Other
Organize meals and snacks within the family	Encourage activity around the home and garden from early life	Set clear maintainable boundaries to behaviour
Eat as a family when possible	Encourage independence in dressing and simple tasks such as bed-making and room tidying	Develop a family policy for the use of television
Promote diets varied in taste and textures	Use leisure time for family to be active together	Develop policies for bedtimes
Encourage home cooking and use of whole foods, fruits and vegetables	Promote active travel to school where practical	Consider lowering the central heating thermostat at home
Avoid adding fats and sugars unnecessarily when preparing or presenting foods: no sugar on the table; unsweetened, unsugared, breakfast cereals; grill rather than fry etc.	Use local play and sports facilities	Encourage children to be self-aware and to understand the benefits of good nutrition and healthy activity
Keep portions modest	Limit time spent in sedentary occupations	Praise and encourage appropriate behaviour to reinforce children's strengths
Do not necessarily expect an empty plate at the end of a meal	Talk with children and help them develop absorbing hobbies	Maintain and improve self-esteem
Develop tactics for dealing with food refusal		Show zero tolerance for bullying tactics of all kinds or for lack of respect for diversity
Avoid compensating food refusal with other favourite foods		
Be circumspect about food 'rewards'		
Use low energy versions of foods when appropriate (see Table 9.6)		
Take note of food labels in relation to high fat, high sugar and total energy content		

Table 13.2. Changes related to eating involved in the weaning process

---

Weaning is a progression from:
- A totally fluid diet to a diet of solids and liquids
- A single food – breast milk or infant formula – to a diet of varied tastes, textures and forms of food
- A liquid diet obtained by sucking to food largely derived by biting and chewing
- Food obtained from breast or bottle to food obtained off a plate with utensils
- Liquids sucked from breast or bottle to those drunk from cup or glass
- Food given to the child to food obtained with own hands or utensils at a communal meal
- Frequent regular feeds to less frequent perhaps less regular meals and occasional small snacks
- Dependency on others for food to ultimately complete control over own diet (a situation which develops long beyond the weaning period as child grows to adult).

It is important that the progression continues with all these items until complete. Children must learn to be confident chewing and to accept varied tastes and textures with foods.

---

weight gain is paralleled by rapid gain in length as very young children set out on trajectories towards tall adult stature. The clue to recognizing this may be in consideration of parental stature.

The potential for physiological fall in %BF during weaning and early childhood is such that the time when non-milk or non-formula foods are first introduced would seem the time when it is most suitable to begin preventive guidance. Many mothers are looking for guidance about the introduction of 'solids' to their infants' diets at this time and are usually ready to listen to advice from professionals. What is introduced to children and practised between parents/carers and children during weaning may be very significant for later dietary habits and lifestyles. The Finnish STRIP study (Hakanen et al. 2006) compared two groups of children followed from 7 months of age. The families (and as they grew older, the children) in the intervention group were given twice yearly counselling on diet and activity. Children's food consumption and activities were documented and discussed with their families in constructive ways so the families could decide for themselves where they might make healthy lifestyle changes. By school age the prevalence of overweight and obesity in the intervention group was significantly less than that in the control group who were reviewed as frequently as the intervention group but given only conventional nurturing advice.

Weaning is a progression (Table 13.2) from a totally fluid diet of breast milk or infant formula to a diet of varied tastes, textures and nutrient density. The progression needs to continue until children are confident chewing a wide range of foods. Parents should not be content to halt the learning to eat process at the stage when the child is happy with soft malleable solids but reluctant to chew. Confidence with chewing some items, for example cooked but unprocessed meat, may take several years. Care may be needed for much longer when young children are eating foods such as apples where choking is a risk if the foods are not chewed sufficiently or are eaten with little attention to the process of chewing.

As the energy content of the solids increases, the energy content of the fluids should decrease by gradually replacing infant formula with dilute juice or water – or providing juice or water instead of some breast feeds. Breast milk volumes usually decline as children take more non-breast-milk foods. Fluids taken from bottles seem comforting to many infants and may be preferred irrespective of their energy content to 'solids'. Developing the balance between drinks and solids is thus not always easy but is usually helped by introducing drinks from cups rather than from bottles at weaning. (Many weanling infants are settled for bed with a bottle of formula long after other drinks are taken from a cup. This may not be very good for dental hygiene but it does seem a comforting way to settle children for sleep. Bottles should be fed before infants are laid down to sleep and should not be left in the cot so the children can suck whilst asleep.)

Young children are very determined

By 7 months old most infants have learnt the skill of shutting their mouths and shaking their heads to indicate 'No'. Food refusal is commonly an indication that the food taste or texture is new and unusual rather than an indication of dislike of that food. It may take 10 to 20 presentations before some foods are accepted (Benton 2004). If parents interpret food refusal too readily as a sign of dislike and thus exclude that food from their children's diets, there is real danger that the children's diets become limited in variety and confined to easy to eat, energy dense, not very satisfying foods (Birch and Fisher 1998). This risks an excess consumption of energy and consequent overweight. Yet, weanlings have real needs both for the micronutrients available from fruits and vegetables and for relatively high energy intakes (for their size) when compared with older children. There is thus a delicate balance between encouraging very young children to eat diets that are varied in nutrient quality and rich in energy, and providing excess energy. Eating at regular meals and organized snacks should help develop appetite and hunger and satiety patterns which enable parents to recognize when their children are satisfied and children to learn hunger/satiety sensations (Birch and Davison 2001).

Young children have very variable appetites

One day they eat very well and then, perhaps the next day, they eat relatively little. What is going on around them during a meal may be more diverting than the process of eating so, with the very young, supervised eating away from disturbing siblings may enable young children to concentrate on eating. If they refuse to eat all that they are offered this may be because they are not hungry. An empty plate should not be seen as an essential conclusion to a meal. However, it may be better to offer small amounts of food with the possibility of second helpings rather than full plates to small children who sometimes seem almost frightened from attempting to eat – to them – huge platefuls of food. If a meal is not finished, appetite for the next meal may be greater provided no snacks are given to compensate for food left uneaten. (There is a remote risk that a small child who has eaten poorly all day could develop nocturnal hypoglycaemia if he or she eats nothing in late afternoon and evening. In such circumstances a drink of infant formula or milk before bed may be advisable.)

Children who are very tired or very hungry may behave very negatively when food is presented. Offering new untried foods to tired children in the expectation that the food will be eaten has a good chance of failure. Whenever possible, avoid leaving mealtimes until children are too tired or too hungry to cooperate.

Weaning may sound simple and straightforward when described here. We recognize that in practice it can be a nightmare in which parents have to compromise over what they hope to achieve for their children's eating behaviours. However, if parents have concepts of what the needs of small children are and how these needs can be met by sound dietary practices, but at the same time develop a sensitivity over how much can be achieved with small children, they may find it easier to surmount some of the difficulties and frustrations which most parents experience from time to time with small children and food. Achieving the ideal healthy diet may be impossible with the vagaries of young children's tastes and appetites but the beginnings of a healthy lifestyle should be encouraged at this age when young children copy and learn very quickly – often with enthusiasm.

Physical activity in young children

It is not just the eating style which can help prevent overweight in the very young (Poskitt 2005). From the earliest age small children should be given opportunities to experience weight bearing activity perhaps initially on rugs on the floor but then in playpens or with toys or carts to push when beginning to get upright. Once walking, small children need opportunities to exercise both within and outside the home. This can involve planned walks and visits to parks and/or playing in the garden. Encouraging imaginative play both in and out of doors, helping children develop skills by involving them in simple ball games, and allowing them to rush around, all contribute to energy expenditure. Indeed one study suggests that small children are awake for such a relatively short period of the day that they have to spend a greater proportion of the day in vigorous energy expenditure than older children and adults if they are to maintain energy balance (Hoos *et al.* 2004). Certainly periods of what appear to adults to be very vigorous activity should be perceived as normal for young children – and should be encouraged in appropriate circumstances although the process of 'growing up' for small children must include learning to control natural exuberance when requested.

Of course small children seem inexhaustible and then suddenly lie down and fall asleep. Or they precipitously decide they are not going to walk any further. If parents have been used to walking and playing with their children they are usually the best judges of when their children are genuinely tired and when they are being negative or simply lazy or looking for the comfort of being carried.

Adolescents

Adolescence has recently been described as 'the most important opportunity to treat emerging problems early and prevent ill-health by educating about and firmly establishing a healthy lifestyle' (Kleinert 2007). We have discussed earlier the difficulties presented by adolescents with overweight/obesity. Peer group eating habits and reduced activity particularly amongst girls make the risk of developing overweight, or of increasing the overweight already present, significant. Further, because of the proximity to adulthood and to the cessation of growth, overweight is more likely to continue into adult life than at earlier ages.

Discussing management of lifestyle issues in relation to adolescence is inevitably hampered by the enormous differences in independence and both physical and psychological maturity of children just entering adolescence and the young adults perhaps leaving home and beginning independent lives sometimes even as parents themselves. This however illustrates the importance of seeing the development of any discussion on behaviour – obesity prevention or any other behaviour – in a changing set-up affected by the individual's own development and by the family environment (Viner and Barker 2005). Adolescents' abilities to choose for themselves must be respected although the extent to which parents and other adults may help them make choices is likely to diminish as the adolescents mature. Adolescents need to be able to find this respect and freedom to choose open to them within health and advisory services as well as within their families (Royal College of General Practitioners/Royal College of Nursing 2002; Royal College of Paediatrics and Child Health 2003).

Dietary habits
Most adolescents are liable to bizarre eating habits from time to time, even if not all the time. Meal skipping, experimental meals concocted by themselves,

'binges' of food either alone or in company with peers, and heavy snacking are some of their many dietary eccentricities (Truswell and Darnton-Hill 1981). Helping adolescents understand the nutrient content of foods, teaching them to cook well, making sure there is always fruit available for snacks and providing them with 'proper' meals when they are at home can be useful home practices to help control excessive energy intakes. Telling adolescents that eating habits or foods are 'bad for them' may be unhelpful in terms of encouraging them to eat well. Pointing out environmental issues in relation to foods – whole foods, organic foods, Fairtrade foods – can be very constructive with some children and may lead to diets richer in whole foods and fruit and unsweetened cereals than before. (The 'food miles' travelled by some fruits at certain times of year may be perceived as negative points! You cannot win all the time!).

Physical activity

Along with support for good diets in adolescence, parents and advisors should tactfully encourage activity since this age group, particularly for girls, is one during which activity levels often drop dramatically. Telling children to be active may not be very helpful, particularly if they are adolescent boys who may feel that all they want to do is spend Saturday mornings in bed. Encouraging some participation in domestic chores – tidying bedroom, preparing and cleaning up after family meals, dog walking and maybe some care of younger siblings – can be helpful if acceptable and should not be devalued by comments such as 'but I did ask you to do that last week'. Suggesting the environmental benefits of walking or cycling rather than going by car, supporting sporting activity by helping with transport to venues (and being prepared to wash muddy sports gear), and similar encouragement of active lifestyles may be a constructive level of parental involvement in adolescent weight control. When adolescents are taking very little exercise it may be worth exploring in sensitive discussion what activity they might enjoy. Schools may find this very helpful when trying to increase activity amongst teenage girls – dancing, aerobics, badminton? – especially if the girls have some choice in the clothing worn for these events.

Schools

The Department of Health (2007a) has produced guidelines on issues relating to childhood overweight and obesity relevant to schools. These build on the main tenets of the Healthy Schools Programme: healthy eating, physical activity, emotional health and well-being, and personal and social health education, but focus on overweight. Current policy is that all children in Reception and Year 6 classes are weighed and measured so changes in the prevalence of overweight/obesity in British children can be documented. The intention is not to label children as overweight nor to fuss the parents that 'something should be done' (Department of Health, 2007b).

Recommendations by the Department of Health (2007a) on matters which might be contributory to reducing the prevalence of childhood overweight/obesity include:

- Ensuring the language and core messages are appropriate:

  Stress positive approaches to overweight management and prevention: be healthy, get active etc.

  Highlight eating a balanced diet rather than pointing out 'good' and 'bad' foods

  Develop the concept of a healthy lifestyle being a lifestyle and not just a diet of healthy food

  Physical activity and an environment which promotes emotional health and well-being must be included within the concept of a healthy lifestyle

  Recognize that PE includes a broad range of activities and not just competitive sport

  Help children understand lifestyle issues so they can make healthy choices for themselves

  Make blame or stigmatization of the overweight/obese unacceptable

- Ensuring universal prevention:

  Adopt school food policies which cover all food/drink brought into schools and not just that provided in tuck shops or at school dinners

  Develop 'engaging' PE curricula which offer opportunities for dancing, aerobics and other individual activities as well as competitive sport

  Encourage children to build their 'physical literacy and personal safety skills' so they and their parents can feel confident about their activity

  Encourage children and their parents and school staff to become involved in healthy lifestyle challenges, for example through getting each individual and family member to identify positive changes they will make each week

- Engaging parents and carers

  Help them understand and support the changes made in school in relation to food and drink

  Encourage community support over presentation and availability of 'healthy' and 'less healthy' foods in shops and food outlets near the school

  Involve parents as much as possible in activity at school and in developing a 'walking school bus' where this seems appropriate. Parents could also become involved in (for example) school gardening projects and cookery demonstrations if these can be timed when parents can attend

  See school–parent activities as opportunities to increase knowledge about the role of diet and activity for health and to advise parents over perceived difficulties in implementing healthier lifestyles

Avoid food rewards in school and discourage these at home

Encourage school (and family) events which are healthy lifestyle challenges.

The Department of Health (2007a) guidance includes many very specific ideas for promoting healthy eating and activity for school populations as part of the Healthy Schools Programme. Currently 86% of schools are involved in the Healthy Schools Programme to some extent. One approach by Hull City Council of offering free 'healthy' school meals to all children (thus avoiding any of the stigma of being a recipient of free school meals) – whilst very expensive – seems to have introduced a high proportion of the school population to eating quality school dinners with some evidence that performance in class has also improved (Colquhoun and Wright 2006).

It is important that all adults, as well as the children, involved with the school demonstrate their own commitment to the principles of healthy lifestyles – or at least appear to do so when on school territory! Children need to see that a healthy lifestyle can be practised and is for life and not something that stops once they escape into the adult world.

There should be key drivers for weight control programmes within the school. One member of staff or a small team of staff and pupils should promote the weight control as well as other healthy lifestyle issues across the school since they can intercalate the – possibly many – suggestions and ideas of other staff and pupils. The drivers also need to develop means of evaluating what is being achieved: what works and what does not work. Without a leading individual or group, enthusiasm may be channelled in too many directions without effective implementation. Or interventions may be restricted to, for example, only one class or year group.

The community

As we have indicated in Chapter 10 there is much that has changed in communities over the past half century that may have contributed to the obesity epidemic particularly by making it less safe, more difficult, or less enjoyable to exercise out of doors both in leisure activities and in physically active travel. A healthy environment will facilitate children being supervised by caring adults, creating low risk of danger from traffic or other environmental hazards, and seeming attractive in terms of facilities offered and the layout of the facilities. Communities should look at their built environment and consider what can be done to make it easier, pleasanter and safer for play and physical activity for all ages (Travers et al. 2006; Alton et al. 2007; Sustrans 2007). In addition there is a need to look for places for activity where adolescents and older children can meet and socialize and be active together other than on the street. Managing youth clubs is not cheap. If youth clubs are to be useful in keeping children and adolescents from loitering on the street they need to be open on a very regular basis. They also need to be attractive places with space for varied activities and for social interaction between peers. If communities are concerned about their young people they may have to lobby local government for support or raise money themselves to improve facilities.

It is difficult to know how much communities should try to influence local trade by encouraging food outlets, particularly those close to schools, to stop promoting energy dense snack items and perhaps promote fruits, vegetables, wholemeal foods and low energy drinks instead. Shopkeepers have to make money to survive and they need to supply what customers want – both those on healthy diets and others. It takes a long time for dietary change across a community – if it occurs at all. Setting up local pressure groups 'For Healthy Diets' equivalent to the Fairtrade movement might encourage shopkeepers to look more critically at what they are selling and possibly change their future promotions.

We have discussed food labelling in Chapter 9. The present system in Britain is confusing since there are two basic approaches, one promoted by the government and one supported by certain food companies. Even for the traffic signal food nutrient signposting scheme promoted by the government, education of the public is needed if the public is to understand the implications of the labels properly (Food Standards Agency 2007). This may be an area where an explanatory leaflet available in places such as doctors' surgeries could be useful or a group teaching session by a practice member or community worker could be held.

What can a primary care trust do to prevent overweight/obesity?

A health centre provides a great opportunity to inform and educate beyond just directing advice at individuals who are perceived as at risk. There are many guidance sheets and recommendations available from both governments and non-governmental organizations concerned with aspects of healthy lifestyles, and other interested parties purveying ideas on the world wide web. Some recommendations may be more suitable in terms of comprehensibility or the quality of advice they offer, than others. The clinic/counselling area/group therapy space should display literature, some perhaps created by the practice so it has a distinct local impact, which provides advice and help on issues relating to weight control in children as well as in adults: diet, activity, lifestyles etc. Some information could be displayed as posters on waiting room walls. Gyms, dance classes, keep fit groups and swimming classes could be listed as well as activities at the local youth club. Practice nurses, health visitors or other interested individuals who have time can arrange sessions in the clinic or some other local area to discuss relevant issues such as food labelling, developing a healthy diet, feeding young children healthily and promoting safe activity. Some practices do have practice walks but these are usually when children are at school and are geared for those adults who may have had medical problems which limit their activity making the walks not suitable for children. Enthusiastic practice members might arrange sessions for teenagers out of school hours, which can involve enjoyable activities relating to developing healthy lifestyles similar to the ideas promoted by MEND and other obesity management groups (Sacher *et al.* 2005). The focus might be particularly at the families with a known history of overweight. However, as we do recognize, the main antagonist to all this is ... lack of time. Are there recently retired practice members who might volunteer to promote healthy lifestyle activities?

There should be named people within the practice from whom advice can be sought. But perhaps the most important aspect is that the prevailing attitude of the practice, clinic or group should be positive, making clear that help can be offered and that there is effective advice and support for overweight children and their families. Overweight is regarded seriously and non-judgementally. Such positive, supportive attitudes should pervade the entire workforce of any clinic, club, group or counselling situation. Ideally, in our equality-in-diversity culture, such attitudes should pervade all society.

In clinical practice the habit of weighing those coming for consultation should be routine. Weighing children must be accompanied by measurement of height since weight alone is more or less meaningless. Weight and height should be plotted on charts and BMI calculated and plotted. If this is done routinely, it is possible to pick up children whose weights are increasing at rates not paralleled by increases in height or whose BMIs are crossing centiles upwards and who are thus at risk of overweight. This opens up opportunities to discuss lifestyles with both children and families.

Government

Of recent years governments in the UK and in other countries have recognized the major problems, both now and for the future, posed by the epidemic of obesity affecting all ages but most concerningly affecting children. This, in the UK, has led to a wealth of documents coming from government and related bodies about the problem and suggesting solutions (See Table 1.4). To some extent there has been help in implementing possible solutions such as through the Free School Fruit Scheme although that scheme has now been more or less subsumed by the promotion of more health related criteria for food in schools and increased subsidies for school meals. Machines selling sweetened, carbonated, brand drinks are no longer present in schools. However, despite all the ideas, papers and recommendations, there seems little effort specifically to support the clinical management of overweight children. There are now many more scientists doing research on childhood obesity and overweight than 20 years ago but the number of paediatricians or paediatric nurses, for example, who run clinical set-ups to manage overweight/obesity in children remains small. Paediatric obesity clinics – even called by less stigmatizing names – remain few and far between. General practitioners who feel confident advising and managing overweight children are also few. Change is needed, especially at the primary care level, since the numbers of overweight and obese – as we have said earlier – are too large for it to be practical to refer all for secondary care. Medical and nursing professionals need to make recommendations to government about what training HCPs need and how many trained HCPs are needed in order to have some impact on the growing prevalence of overweight in childhood. How much can schoolteachers also be encouraged to spare time to learn about childhood overweight/obesity so that they can incorporate healthy lifestyle promotion within curricula? All this may seem idealistic given the full days of most HCPs and teachers but without committed individuals it is going to be difficult to create the ambience in which to build healthy lifestyles and have an impact on the rise in childhood obesity and overweight.

Industry

The food industry takes a lot of flak for the prevalence of overweight/obesity today – with some justification. We cannot show that the obese routinely eat more than the non-obese so we cannot put all the blame on industry. Nevertheless it is infinitely easier to obtain an excess of calories in most industrialized countries today than it was 50 years ago. Portion sizes of many food items have increased for what we must presume are commercial reasons since we know of no one who complained that the size of muffins in the past was too small; that there were not enough biscuits in the snack pack; or that French breadstick sandwiches were too short. Yet increased portion sizes mean we not only pay more for food items but – assuming we eat all the item – we consume more energy without necessarily planning to do so (Rolls *et al.* 2006). In many cases fat and sugar are added unnecessarily to food items – either as integral components or as topping or decoration – and the energy contents of foods increase.

Some supermarkets have recognized that many of the public are interested in obtaining less energy dense foods. They have introduced low energy versions of some items and promotions of 'healthy' foods. Parents and community members need to realize that they, the purchasers, have the power to get food manufacturers to change what they provide.

Where there has been real concern about the health of a population, focused efforts by whole communities supported by governments can make very significant changes. The way in which heart disease and hyperlipidaemia have been reduced in Finland is a splendid example of how a population's habits can be changed for the benefit of many (Hakanen *et al.* 2006). We need to work towards focused programmes for childhood obesity too but efforts towards these tend to come up against comments such as 'It is the individual's choice' and 'Beware the nanny state'. This is sad since individuals and communities need support to change (Avenell *et al.* 2006). (Also, many nannies were very skilled at helping children make good choices.) Help and support may be especially needed in those areas where deprivation, food deserts and low educational levels make it more difficult for communities to feel sufficiently empowered to change their lifestyles. Yet it is often families in these areas who are most at risk of childhood and adult overweight and the complications that go with overweight.

Commercial promotion

Snack items are now widely promoted in a variety of packaging and flavours so consumers, especially children, are encouraged to collect wrappers or try out the different tastes thus sampling more than one of each item or sampling too frequently. Studies show that satiety for a particular item (such as potato crisps) is less if different flavours of the item are consumed rather than if only items of one flavour are consumed. Controls on advertising need to discourage the variety in packaging and packaging several items together or 'two for the price of one' all of which seem likely to encourage over consumption of specific foods. A parent may buy a 'bumper' pack and put all except one item aside for another occasion but will a child buying the same 'bumper' pack do this?

The media

We have discussed the importance of developing family policies for television viewing in the management of overweight/obesity. Family policies which limit television viewing are very relevant in the prevention of overweight as well. The extent to which increased television viewing has contributed to the increase in overweight children is not clear but, in very general terms, the increase seems to parallel the rise in available viewing hours and the range of programmes available rather well (Gortmaker *et al.* 1996).

It is not just the sedentariness of viewing which affects weight control but the effects of advertisements on television which act to promote overweight. The Hastings Report (Hastings *et al.* 2003) concluded that there was a lot of food advertising to children; the advertised diet was less healthy than the recommended one; children enjoy and engage with food promotion; food promotion has an effect on children's preferences, purchasing behaviour and consumption; and these effects are independent of other factors and operating at both brand and category levels.

Ofcom (Office of Communications) has recently made public its policies for advertising and children on television (Ofcom 2007). From April 2007, products classified as HFSS (high fat, high sugar or high salt) by the FSA cannot be used in sponsorship or advertising in and around programmes thought to appeal to children 4–9 years old. From January 2008 this restriction shall be extended to all programmes which might appeal to children under 16 years. The use of celebrities shall also be prohibited in advertising for these products. Some feel these regulations do not go far enough and would prefer the ban include all programmes before the 9 pm 'watershed'. The situation will be reviewed in 2008.

The media present enormous potential for the promotion of healthy living. This creates considerable responsibilities in this area. What is likely to be perceived as a programme of lifestyle recommendations, particularly when dealing with diet where eccentric ideas often blossom, should come from qualified professionals with balanced nutritional and health views and not from those with views recognized as extreme or eccentric. Eccentric hypotheses can make enthralling television since challenging authority and accepted dogma can be welcomed by our rather over-critical-of-authority society. However most viewers/listeners are not in the position to evaluate the science behind an idea for themselves. This needs remembering and the relative value, in terms of scientific acceptance, of lifestyles portrayed on television, even as documentaries, should be made clear.

What can television and other media do to help prevent overweight (other than control advertising of HFSS foods)? We do not suggest that programmes turn over entirely to high-minded proponents of healthy lifestyles but a scattering of programmes that are educative and promotional for better lifestyles and for training children in healthy behaviours could be very helpful and can be made interesting.

Thus:

- Present 'out of doors' in a more positive light to young people. Too often television portrays the world outside the home as populated by pollutants, dangerous traffic and even more dangerous strangers.
- Provide entertaining programmes, at times when children may be watching, which encourage activity, e.g. imitation of dancing/movement on the screen in association with music
- Present children's gardening and vegetable growing advice with guidance on growing foodstuffs in pots for those with no garden space.
- Present programmes with simple nutritional and health advice suitable for children.
- Develop cookery programmes geared for children which introduce relatively low fat, low sugar, tasty items that children can prepare safely at home.

- Encourage activity through programmes educating children about less familiar games and sports.
- Make sure bullying, if portrayed at all, is never glorified. Make programmes 'weight-blind' and celebrating diversity.
- Develop regular local programmes which present interesting walks, natural history, potentially active days out for the family.
- Use funds to promote charities supporting environmental improvement and opportunities for children.

Many of these things already happen but perhaps they need to be promoted to more peak viewing times or be more widespread.

What is the role of the health care professional in community change?

We have already discussed what can be done within a primary care set-up. But HCPs have wider responsibilities. As members of the community who have some understanding of what is required to promote healthy living they should see themselves as role models for healthy living and as advocates of positive lifestyle change. They can set examples – which do not have to be extreme but could include doing things such as using stairs for journeys up only a few flights; walking or cycling or taking a bus rather than using a car when time and work permit; eating plenty of fruit and vegetables and encouraging the same within their families; reducing snacking ... etc.

Current interest in global warming and the damage modern society is causing the environment stresses the need for actions which, in many cases, will also benefit nutritional health. Reducing the use of cars and polluting transports in favour of walking and cycling, supporting the development of woods and parks, eating locally grown foods including fruits and vegetables, and reducing the heating within the home are lifestyle changes which can promote weight control as well as reduce individual 'carbon footprints'. Similarly, policies for cardiac health and reducing the risk of cancer involve dietary, activity and weight changes similar to those which promote overweight prevention. Thus programmes do not need to be developed specifically for obesity prevention but for the non-specific promotion of sustainable healthy living for families and communities.

In addition to promoting healthy living by acting as role models, HCPs should also consider how they can effect community change. Lobbying locally for change in green spaces and transport and improvement in many facilities should be considered another possible area of responsibility (Larkin 2003). Working with individuals in the community gives HCPs a particular insight into what are the real barriers to implementing change for the individual or within families and schools.

Evaluation

Families who are concerned that their children may be developing overweight often also recognize when their children are successfully controlling their weight. If the family is one with a history of overweight this can readily be accepted as the consequence of efforts to develop healthy behaviours. The effects of anti-obesity programmes on populations – nations or communities – are less easy to assess. Yet we need to be able to evaluate the effectiveness, particularly the cost-effectiveness, of initiatives.

Clinic and school weight, height and BMI records are one way of assessing the effect of initiatives to reduce the incidence of childhood overweight. Regular FFQs documenting high energy snacks versus fresh fruit and vegetable consumption (for example) can be used to document changes in the diets of communities but will not directly document population weight changes. Data collected by non-governmental organizations interested in active travel, such as the cycling promoting organization Sustrans (2007), and by the Department for Transport can indicate whether there are significant positive changes in the use of transport. Memberships of sports and gym clubs by young people are other data which could contribute to documenting relevant changes. All these methods are very limited in the information they provide although added together they could indicate significant changes in prevailing attitudes within communities. We do need good objective methods of assessing lifestyle changes and of relating these to changes in documented BMIs for age. If there is no evidence of changing prevalence of overweight, is this because programmes have not been evaluated long enough or are the programmes not reaching the most at risk or are they simply ineffective and in need of change? If a programme is not working – has it been implemented properly? Has it had any effect at all? How quickly can we expect to see population changes? Nationwide and worldwide there are many projects running and plenty of good ideas for action to prevent childhood overweight and obesity. But programmes need evaluation and sound research evaluations need spreading out into communities and their implications discussed. The nutritional fate of today's young children cannot wait whilst society muddles along with projects and programmes which years later turn out to be ineffective. If something is not working, at the least some aspects need changing. Evaluations need to be ongoing. Healthy lifestyle promotion needs implementing, evaluating, modifying and reassessing until success is achieved. Then successful programmes for sustainable healthy lifestyles need embedding in child-rearing practices so we can begin to undermine the present unremitting rise in childhood overweight.

Recommendations

- Obesity prevention measures within the home are similar to the obesity management measures described in much of this book and may be effective with a slightly 'lighter touch'.
- Weaning and adolescence are ages when diet and activity are critical periods for learning healthy behaviours. Healthy practices that can be sustained into later life should be encouraged.
- Communities can do much to improve the local environment in ways that will benefit health – and help prevent obesity in the process: joined-up public transport; cycle tracks; safe footpaths; play areas, playing fields and youth clubs which are supervised, safe and attractive.
- Schools have a significant role in the prevention of overweight if they are allowed to devote the necessary time to educate and implement advice on activity and food availability, perhaps supported through the Healthy Schools Programme.
- Local food outlets and major supermarkets have a significant role in reducing the promotion of HFSS foods; using understandable food labelling systems which indicate energy dense, HFSS foods; making fresh fruit and vegetables available at affordable prices; providing low energy versions of traditional foods.
- Governments have a major role in warning the public of the risks of pursuing certain lifestyles.
- Governments need to facilitate overweight prevention through encouraging and financially supporting facilities and training for professionals who are trying to manage and prevent overweight.
- Those concerned with childhood overweight need to recognize they will be seen as role models and advocates for positive change.

References

Adam-Perrot, A., Clifton, P., Brouns, F., 2006. Low-carbohydrate diets: nutritional and physiological aspects. *Obes. Rev.*, **7**, 49–58.

Ainsworth, B. E., Haskell, W. L., Whitt, M. C., Irwin, M. L., Swartz, A. M., Strath, S. J., O'Brien, W. L., Bassett, D. R. Jr, Schmitz, K. H., Emplaincourt, P. O., Jacobs, D. R. Jr, Leon, A. S., 2000. Compendium of physical activities: an update of activity codes and MET intensities. *Med. Sci. Sports Exerc.*, **32**, S498–504.

Alberti, G. K., Zimmet, P., Shaw, J., IDF Epidemiology Task Force Consensus Group, 2005. The metabolic syndrome: a new worldwide definition. *Lancet*, **366**, 1059–62.

Alton, D., Adab, P., Roberts, L., Barrett, T., 2007. Relationship between walking levels and perceptions of the local neighbourhood environment. *Arch. Dis. Child.*, **92**, 29–33.

Alvina, M., Araya, H., 2004. Rapid carbohydrate digestion rate produced lesser short term satiety in obese preschool children. *Eur. J. Clin. Nutr.*, **58**, 637–42.

American Thoracic Society, 1999. Cardiorespiratory sleep studies in children. *Am. J. Respir. Crit. Care Med.*, **160**, 1381–7.

Anderson, A. S., 2002. Lifestyle interventions: how joined up are we? *J. Hum. Nutr. Diet*, **15**, 241–2.

Araujo, C. L., Victoria, C. G., Hallal, P. C., Gigante, D. P., 2006. Breast feeding and overweight in childhood: evidence from the Pelotas 1993 birth cohort study. *Int. J. Obes.*, **30**, 500–6.

Armstrong, N., Balding, J., Gentle, P., Kirby, B., 1990. Patterns of physical activity among 11 to 16 year old British children. *Br. Med. J.*, **301**, 203–5.

Armstrong, J., Dorosty, A. R., Reilly, J. J., Child Health Information Team, Emmett, P. M., 2003. Coexistence of social inequalities in undernutrition and obesity in preschool children: population based cross sectional study. *Arch. Dis. Child.*, **88**, 671–5.

Astrup, A., 2006. Have we been barking up the wrong tree: can a good night's sleep make us slimmer? *Int. J. Obes.*, **30**, 1025–6.

Augustin, L. S., Francechi, S., Jenkins, D. J. A., Kendall, C. W. C., La Vecchia, C., 2002. Glycemic index in chronic disease: a review. *Eur. J. Clin. Nutr.*, **556**, 1049–71.

Avenell, A., Sattar, N., Lean, M., 2006. Management: Part 1 – Behaviour change, diet and activity. *Br. Med. J.*, **333**, 740–3.

Baird, J., Fisher, D., Lucas, P., Kleijnen, J., Roberts, H., Law, C., 2005. Being big or growing fast: systematic review of size and growth in infancy and later obesity. *Br. Med. J.*, **331**, 929–31.

Barker, D. J. P., 1994. *Mothers, Babies and Disease in later life*. London: BMJ Press.

Beevers, G., Lip, G. Y. H., O'Brien, P. E., 2001. Blood pressure measurement: Part II – Conventional sphygmomanometry: technique of auscultatory blood pressure measurement. *Br. Med. J.*, **322**, 1043–7.

Belamarich, P. F., Luder, E., Kattan, M., Mitchell, H., Islam, S., Lynn, H., Crain, E. F., 2000. Do obese inner-city children with asthma have more symptoms than nonobese children with asthma? *Pediatrics*, **106**, 1436–41.

Benton, D., 2004. Role of parents in the determination of the food preferences of children and the development of obesity. *Int. J. Obes.*, **28**, 858–69.

Bergmann, K. E., Bergmann, R. L., von Kries, R., Böhm, O., Richter, R., Dudenhausen, J. W., Wahn, U., 2003. Early determinants of childhood overweight and adiposity in a birth cohort study: risk of breast feeding. *Int. J. Obes.*, **27**, 162–72.

Biddle, S. J., Gorely, T., Stensel, D. J., 2004. Health-enhancing physical activity and sedentary behaviour in children and adolescents. *J. Sports Sci.*, **22**, 679–01.

Birch, L. L., Davison, K. K., 2001. Family environmental factors influencing the developing behavioral controls of food intake and childhood overweight. *Pediatr. Clin. North Am.*, **48**, 893–907.

Birch, L. L., Fisher, J. O., 1998. Development of eating behaviours among children and adolescents. *Pediatrics*, **101**, 539–49.

Bjorntorp, P., 2001. Thrifty genes and human obesity: are we chasing ghosts? *Lancet*, **358**, 1006–8.

Bodurtha, J. N., Mosteller, M., Hewitt, J. K., Nance, W. E., Eaves, L. J., Moskowitz, W. B., Katz, S., Schicken, R. M., 1990. Genetic analysis of anthropometric measures in 11-year-old twins: the Medical College of Virginia Twin Study. *Pediatr. Res.*, **28**, 1–4.

Bogardus, C., Lillioja, S., Ravussin, E., Abbott, W., Zawadzki, J. K., Young, A., Knowler, W. C., Jacobowitz, R., Moll, P. P., 1986. Familial dependency of resting metabolic rate. *New Engl. J. Med.*, **315**, 96–100.

Bogin, B., 1999. *Patterns of Human Growth*, 2nd edn. Cambridge, UK: Cambridge University Press.

Børjeson, M., 1976. The aetiology of obesity in children: a study of 101 twin pairs. *Acta Paediatr. Scand.*, **65**, 279–87.

Bouchard, C., Tremblay, A., Després, J.-P., Nadeau, A., Lupein, P. J., Thériault, G., Dussault, J., Moorjani, S., Pinault, S., Fournier, G., 1990. The response to long term overfeeding in identical twins. *New Engl. J. Med.*, **322**, 1477–82.

Brambilla, P., Bedogni, G., Moreno, L. A., Goran, M. I., Gutin, B., Fox, K. R., Peters, D. M., Barbeau, P., De Simone, M., Pietrobelli, A., 2006. Crossvalidation of anthropometry against magnetic resonance imaging for the assessment of visceral and subcutaneous adipose tissue in children. *Int. J. Obes.*, **30**, 23–30.

British Nutrition Foundation, 1999. *Obesity: Report of the British Nutrition Task Force*. Oxford, UK: Blackwell Scientific.

Broom, J., Haslam, D., 2004. Programme to fight obesity already exists. *Br. Med. J.*, **329**, 53.

Broom, J., Reckless, J., Kumar, S., Lean, M., Frost, G., Barth, J., Finer, N., Haslam, D., Pearson, D., Campbell, I., Wayne, C., Banks, I., Deville-Almond, J., Stott, R., Ali, O., 2004. Fighting obesity in primary care. *Br. Med. J.*, **328**, 1327.

Brummer, E., McCarthy, N., 2001. Adult obesity depends on genes and environment. *Br. Med. J.*, **323**, 52.

Buggs, C., Rosenfield, R.L., 2005. Polycystic ovary syndrome in adolescence. *Endocrinol. Metab. Clin. North Am.*, **34**, 677–705.

Burdette, H.L., Whitaker, R.C., Hall, W.C., Daniels, S.R., 2006. Breastfeeding, introduction of complementary foods and adiposity at 5y of age. *Am. J. Clin. Nutr.*, **83**, 550–8.

Burke, V., Beilin, L.J., Simmer, K., Oddy, W.H., Blake, K.V., Doherty, D., Kendall, G.E., Newnham, J.P., Landau, L.I., Stanley, F.J., 2005. Predictors of body mass index and associations with cardiovascular risk factors in Australian children: a prospective cohort study. *Int. J. Obes.*, **29**, 15–23.

Cade, J., Thompson, R., Burley, V., Warm, D., 2002. Development, validation and utilization of food-frequency questionnaires: a review. *Publ. Hlth Nutr.*, **5**, 467–87.

Carrel, A.L., Moerchen, V., Myers, S.E., Bekx, M.T., Whitman, B.Y., Allen, D.B., 2004. Growth hormone improves mobility and body composition in infants and toddlers with Prader–Willi syndrome. *J. Pediatr.*, **145**, 744–9.

Carskadon, M.A., Acebo, C., Jenni, O.G., 2004. Regulation of adolescent sleep: implications for behavior. *Ann. N. Y. Acad. Sci.*, **1021**, 292–3.

Chaput, J-P., Brunet, M., Tremblay, A., 2006. Relationship between short sleeping hours and childhood overweight/obesity: results from the 'Québec en forme' project. *Int. J. Obes.*, **30**, 1080–5.

Charles, M.A., Eschwege, E., Grandmottet, P., Isnard, F., Cohen, J.M., Bensoussan, J.L., Berche, H., Chapiro, O., Andre, P., Vague, P., Juhan-Vague, I., Bard, J.M., Safar, M., 2000. Treatment with metformin of non-diabetic men with hypertension, hypertriglyceridaemia and central fat distribution: the BIGPRO 1.2 trial. *Diabetes*, **23**, 26–32.

Chief Medical Officer Report, 2004. *At Least Five a Week: Evidence on the Impact of Physical Activity and its Relationship to Health.* London: HMSO.

Child Growth Foundation, 2007. BMI Chart 0–20 Years. London: Child Growth Foundation. Available online at www.childgrowthfoundation.org

Chinn, S., Rona, R.J., 2001. International definition of overweight and obesity for children: a lasting solution? *Ann. Hum. Biol.*, **29**, 306–13.

Clark, H.R., Goyder, E., Bissell, P., Blank, L., Peters, J., 2007. How do parents' child-feeding behaviours influence child weight? Implications for childhood obesity policy. *J. Publ. Hlth*, **10**, 1093/pubmed/fdm012

Cleland, V., Venn, A., Fryer, J., Dwyer, J., Blizzard, L., 2005. Parental exercise is associated with Australian children's extracurricular sports participation and cardiorespiratory fitness: a cross-sectional study. *Int. J. Behav. Nutr. Phys. Act.*, **2**, 3–11.

Clifford, T.J., 2003. Breast feeding and obesity. *Br. Med. J.*, **327**, 879–80.

Cole, T.J., Freeman, J.V., Preece, M.A., 1995. Body mass index reference curves for the UK, 1990. *Arch. Dis. Child.*, **73**, 25–9.

Cole, T.J., Bellizzi, M.C., Flegal, K.M., Dietz, W.H., 2000. Establishing a standard definition for child overweight and obesity worldwide: international survey. *Br. Med. J.*, **320**, 1240.

Colquhoun, D., Wright, N., 2006. *Free Healthy School Meals.* Available online at www.hull.ac.uk/ces/resourcesandconsultancy/FreeHealthySchoolMeals.html

Cooke, L. J., Wardle, J., Gibson, E. L., Spochnik, M., Sheiham, A., Lawson, M., 2004. Demographic, familial and trait predictors of fruit and vegetable consumption by pre-school children. *Publ. Hlth Nutr.,* **7**, 251–2.

Coon, K. A., Tucker, K. L., 2002. Television and children's consumption patterns: a review of the literature. *Min. Pediatr.,* **54**, 423–36.

Coon, K. A., Goldberg, J., Rogers, B. L., Tucker, K. L., 2001. Relationship between use of television during meals and children's food consumption patterns. *Pediatrics,* **107**, 1/e7.

Cooper, A. R., Anderson, L. B., Wedderkopp, N., Page, A. S., Froberg, K., 2005. Physical activity levels of children who walk, cycle or are driven to school. *Am. J. Prev. Med.,* **29**, 179–84.

Cooper, T. V., Klesges, L. M., Debon, M., Klesges, R. C., Shelton, M. L., 2006. An assessment of obese and non obese girls' metabolic rate during television viewing, reading and resting. *Eat. Behav.,* **7**, 105–14.

Counterweight Project Team, 2004. Current approaches to obesity management in UK primary care: the Counterweight Programme. *J. Hum. Nutr. Dietet.,* **17**, 183–90.

Cruz, M. L., Goran, M. I., 2004. The metabolic syndrome in children and adolescents. *Curr. Diabet. Rep.,* **4**, 53–62.

Cutting, T. A., Fisher, J. O., Grimm-Thomas, K., Birch, L. L., 1999. Like mother, like daughter: familial patterns of overweight are mediated by mothers' dietary disinhibition. *Am. J. Clin. Nutr.,* **69**, 608–13.

Davies, P. S., Evans, S., Broomhead, S., Clough, H., Day, J. M., Laidlaw, A., Barnes, N. D., 1998. Effect of growth hormone on height, weight and body composition in Prader–Willi syndrome. *Arch. Dis. Child.,* **78**, 474–6.

Davison, K. K., Lawson, C. T., 2006. Do attributes in the physical environment influence children's physical activity? A review of the literature. *Int. J. Behav. Nutr. Phys. Act.,* **3**, 19–37.

de Castro, J. M., 1996. How can eating behavior be regulated in the complex environments of free-living humans. *Neurosci. Biol. Rev.,* **20**, 119–31.

Deane, S., Thomson, A., 2006. Obesity and the pulmonologist. *Arch. Dis. Child.,* **91**, 188–191.

Department of Health, 2004. *Choosing Health.* London: The Stationery Office. Available online at www.dh.gov.uk/PublicationsAndStatistics

Department of Health, 2007a. *Obesity Guidance for Healthy Schools Coordinators and their Partners.* London: The Stationery Office. Available online at www.library.nhs.uk/guidelinesFinder/viewResource

Department of Health, 2007b. *Supporting Healthy Lifestyles: The National Child Measurement Programme – Guidance for the School Year 2006–7.* London: The Stationery Office. Available online at www.dh.gov.uk

Department for Transport, 2002. *Cycling in Great Britain.* London: The Stationery Office.

Department for Transport, 2007. *Cycling Personal Travel Sheet.* London: The Stationery Office. Available online at www.dft.gov.uk/transtat

Dietz, W. H., 1994. Critical periods in childhood for the development of obesity. *Am. J. Clin. Nutr.,* **59**, 955–9.

Dietz, W. H., 1998. Health consequences of obesity in youth: childhood predictors of adult disease. *Pediatrics*, **101**, 518–25.

Dietz, W. H., 2001. The obesity epidemic in young children: reduce television viewing and promote playing. *Br. Med. J.*, **322**, 313–14.

Dietz, W. H., Gortmaker, S. L., 1985. Do we fatten our children in front of the television set: obesity and television viewing in children and adolescents. *Pediatrics*, **75**, 805–812.

Dietz, W. H., Gross, W. L., Kirkpatrick, J. A., 1982. Blount disease (tibia vara): another skeletal disorder associated with childhood obesity. *J. Pediatr.*, **101**, 735–7.

Dixon-Woods, M., Young, B., Heney, D., 1999. Partnerships with children. *Br. Med. J.*, **319**, 778–80.

Drake, A. J., Smith, A., Betts, P. R., Crowne, E. C., Shield, J. P., 2002. Type 2 diabetes in obese white children. *Arch. Dis. Child.*, **86**, 207–8.

Eckel, R. H., Grundy, S. M., Zimmet, P. Z., 2005. The metabolic syndrome. *Lancet*, **365**, 1415–28.

Edmunds, L. D., 2005. Parents' perceptions of health professionals' responses when seeking help for their overweight children. *Fam. Pract.*, **22**, 287–92.

Edmunds, L. D., Waters, E., 2004. Childhood obesity. In *Evidence Based Pediatrics and Child Health*, 2nd edn, ed. V. A. Moyer, E. Elliot, R. Gilbert, T. Klassen, S. Logan, C. Mellis, D. J. Henderson-Smart, K. Williams, pp. 223–39. London: BMJ Press.

Edmunds, L., Waters, E., Elliott, E. J., 2001. Evidence based management of childhood obesity. *Br. Med. J.*, **323**, 916–9.

Edmunds, L. D., Rudolf, M. C. J., Mulley, B., 2007. How should we tackle obesity in the really young? *Arch. Dis. Child.*, **92** (Suppl. 1) A75.

Edwards, C., Nicholls, D., Croker, H., VanZyl, S., Viner, R., Wardle, J., 2006. Family-based behavioural treatment of obesity: acceptability and effectiveness in the UK. *Eur. J. Clin. Nutr.*, **60**, 587–92.

Ehtisham, S., Barrett, T., 2003. The emergence of type 2 diabetes in childhood: diagnosis, management and outlook. *Mod. Diabet. Managemt.*, **4**, 2–6.

Ehtisham, S., Hattersley, A. T., Dunger, D. B., Barrett, T. G., 2004. First UK survey of paediatric type 2 diabetes and MODY. *Arch. Dis. Child.*, **89**, 526–9.

Eiholzer, U., Whitman, B. Y., 2004. A comprehensive team approach to the management of patients with Prader–Willi syndrome. *J. Pediatr. Endocrinol. Metab.*, **17**, 1153–75.

Eiholzer, U., Nordmann, Y., l'Allemand, D., Schlumpf, M., Schmid, S., Kromeyer-Hauschild, K., 2003. Improving body composition and physical activity in Prader–Willi syndrome. *J. Pediatr.*, **142**, 73–8.

Ekaitis, B., 2007. A Prader–Willi food pyramid. Available online at www.pwsausa.org/syndrome/foodpyramid.htm

Epstein, L. H., Wing, R. R., Penner, B. C., Kress, M. J., 1985. Effect of diet and controlled exercise on weight loss in obese children. *J. Pediatr.*, **107**, 358–61.

Epstein, L. H., Myers, M. D., Raynor, H. A., Saelens, B. E., 1998. Treatment of pediatric obesity. *Pediatrics*, **101**, 554–70.

Eriksson, J. G., Forsen, T., Tuomilehto, J., Winter, P. D., Osmond, C., Barker, D. J., 1999. Catch-up growth in childhood and death from coronary heart disease: longitudinal study. *Br. Med. J.*, **318**, 427–31.

Eston, R. G., Brodie, D. A., Mist, B. A., Poskitt, E. M. E., 1990. Cardiorespiratory responses to cycle ergometry in obese and normal children. In *Children and Exercise, 14th International Seminar of Pediatric Work Physiology*, ed. G. Buenen, J. Ghesquiers, T. Reybrouk, A. L. Claessens, p. 114. Stuttgart, Germany: Ferdinand Enke.

Evenson, K. R., Birnbaum, A. S., Bedimo-Rung, A. L., Sallis, J. F., Voorhees, C. C., Ring, K., Elder, J. P., 2006. Girls' perception of physical environmental factors and transportation: reliability and association with physical activity and active transport to school. *Int. J. Behav. Nutr. Phys. Act.*, **3**, 28–43.

Fallowfield, L., Jenkins, V., 2004. Communicating sad, bad, and difficult news in medicine. *Lancet*, **363**, 312–19.

Farooqi, I. S., O'Rahilly, S., 2000. Recent advances in the genetics of severe childhood obesity. *Arch. Dis. Child.*, **83**, 31–4.

Fields, D. A., Goran, M. I., McCrory, M. A., 2002. Body composition assessment in adults and children: a review. *Am. J. Clin. Nutr.*, **75**, 453–67.

Fitness Canada, 1981. *Standardized Test of Fitness: Operations Manual*, 2nd edn. Ottawa, ON: Ministry of Fitness and Amateur Sport.

Flodmark, C. E., Ohlsson, T., Ryden, O., Sveger, T., 1993. Prevention of progression to severe obesity in a group of obese schoolchildren treated with family therapy. *Pediatrics*, **91**, 880–4.

Fomon, S. J., 1974. *Infant Nutrition.* Philadelphia, PA: W.B. Saunders.

Food Standards Agency, 2007. *Signposting: Traffic Light Labelling.* London: The Stationery Office. Available online at www.eatwell.gov.uk

Forster, J. L., Gourash, L. M., 2005. *Managing Prader–Willi Syndrome: A Primer for Psychiatrists.* Available online at www.pwsausa.org

Foster, G. D., Makris, A. P., Bailer, B. A., 2005. Behavioral treatment of obesity. *Am. J. Clin. Nutr.*, **82**, 230S–235S.

Fox, K. R., Edmunds, L. D., 2000. Growing up as a 'fat kid': can schools help provide a better experience? *J. Emot. Behav. Prob.*, **9**, 177–81.

Franklin, J., Denyer, G., Steinbeck, K. S., Caterson, I. D., Hill, A. J., 2006. Obesity and risk of low self-esteem: a statewide survey of Australian children. *Pediatrics*, **118**, 2481–7.

Freedman, D. S., Khan, L. K., Serdula, M. K., Dietz, W. H., Srinivasan, S. R., Berensen, G. S., 2003. The relation of menarcheal age to obesity in childhood and adulthood. *BMC Paediatr*, **3**, e3.

Freeman, J. V., Cole, T. J., Chinn, S., Jones, P. R., White, E. M., Preece, M. A., 1995. Cross sectional stature and weight reference curves for the UK, 1990. *Arch. Dis. Child.*, **73**, 17–24.

Freemark, M., Bursey, D., 2001. The effects of metformin on body mass index and glucose tolerance in obese adolescents with fasting hyperinsulinaemia and a family history of type 2 diabetes. *Pediatrics*, **107**, e55.

Frelut, M-L., 2002. Interdisciplinary residential management. In *Child and Adolescent Obesity*, ed. W. Burniat, T. Cole, I. Lissau, E. Poskitt, pp. 377–88. Cambridge, UK: Cambridge University Press.

French, S. A., Story, M., Perry, C. L., 1995. Self-esteem and obesity in children and adolescents: a literature review. *Obes. Res.*, **3**, 479–90.

Garcia, V. F., DeMaria, E. J., 2006. Adolescent bariatric surgery: treatment delayed, treatment denied, a crisis invited. *Obes. Surg.*, **16**, 1–4.

Garn, S. M., 1976. The origins of obesity. *Am. J. Dis. Child.*, **130**, 465–7.

Garn, S. M., Lavelle, M., 1985. Two decade follow-up of fatness in early childhood. *Am. J. Dis. Child.*, **139**, 465–7.

Garrow, J., 2005. Body size and composition. In *Human Nutrition* 11th edn, ed. C. A. Geissler, H. J. Powers, pp. 65–82. Edinburgh, UK: Elsevier.

Gately, P. J., Cooke, C. B., Barth, J. H., Bewick, B. M., Radley, D., Hill, A. J., 2005. Children's residential weight-loss programs can work: a prospective cohort study of short-term outcomes for overweight and obese children. *Pediatrics*, **116**, 73–7.

Gehling, R. K., Magarey, A. M., Daniels, L. A., 2005. Food based recommendations to reduce fat intake: an evidence based approach to the development of a family-focused child weight management programme. *J. Paediatr. Child Hlth*, **41**, 112–18.

Golley, R. K., Magarey, A. M., Steinbeck, K. S., Baur, L. A., Daniels, L. A., 2006. Comparison of metabolic syndrome prevalence using six different definitions in overweight pre-pubertal children enrolled in a weight management study. *Int. J. Obes.*, **30**, 853–60.

Goodman, E., Whitaker, R. C., 2002. A prospective study of the role of depression in the development and persistence of adolescent obesity. *Pediatrics*, **109**, 497–504.

Golan, M., Crow, S., 2004. Targeting parents exclusively in the treatment of childhood obesity: long-term results. *Obes. Res.*, **12**, 357–61.

Goran, M. I., 1998. Measurement issues related to studies of childhood obesity: assessment of body composition, body fat distribution, physical activity, and food intake. *Pediatrics*, **101**, 505–19.

Gortmaker, S. L., Must, A., Sobol, A. M., Peterson, K., Colditz, G. A., Dietz, W. H., 1996. Television viewing as a cause of increasing obesity among children in the United States, 1986–1990. *Arch. Pediatr. Adolesc. Med.*, **150**, 356–62.

Gregory, J. R., Lowe, S., 2000. *National Diet and Nutrition Survey: Young People Aged 4–18 Years*, vol. 1, *Report of the Diet and Nutrition Survey*. London: The Stationery Office.

Gregory, J. R., Collins, D. L., Davies, P. S. W., Hughes, J. M., Clarke P. C., *et al.*, 1995. *National Diet and Nutrition Survey: Children Aged $1\frac{1}{2} - 4\frac{1}{2}$ years*, vol. 1, *Report of the Diet and Nutrition Survey*. London: The Stationery Office.

Griffiths, L. J., Wolke, D., Page, A. S., Horwood, J. P., the ALSPAC Study Team, 2006. Obesity and bullying: different effects for boys and girls. *Arch. Dis. Child.*, **91**, 121–5.

Griffiths, M., Payne, P. R., 1976. Energy expenditure in small children of obese and non-obese parents. *Nature*, **260**, 698–700.

Grund, A., Krause, H., Siewers, M., Rieckert, H., Muller, M. J., 2001. Is TV viewing an index of physical activity and fitness in overweight and normal weight children? *Publ. Hlth. Nutr.*, **4**, 1245–51.

Gunay-Aygun, M., Schwartz, S., Heeger, S., O'Riordan, M. A., Cassidy, S. B., 2001. The changing purpose of Prader–Willi syndrome clinical diagnostic criteria and proposed revised criteria. *Pediatrics*, **108**, e92.

Haby, M. M., Vos, T., Carter, R., Moodie, M., Markwick, A., Magnus, A., Tay-Teo, K. S., Swinburn, B., 2006. A new approach to assessing the health benefit from obesity interventions in children and adolescents: the Assessing Cost-effectiveness in Obesity Project. *Int. J. Obes.*, **30**, 1463–75.

Hakanen, M., Lagstrom, H., Kaitosaari, T., Niinikoski, H., Nanto-Salonen, K., Jokinen, E., Sillanmaki, L., Viikari, J., Ronnemaa, T., Simell, O., 2006. Development of overweight in an atherosclerosis prevention trial starting in early childhood: the STRIP study. *Int. J. Obes.*, **30**, 618–26.

Hales, C. N., Barker, D. J. P., 1992. Non-insulin dependent (type II) diabetes mellitus: thrifty phenotype hypothesis. In *Fetal and Infant Origins of Adult Disease*, ed. D. J. P. Barker, pp. 258–72. London: BMJ Press.

Hancox, R. J., Poulton, R., 2006. Watching television is associated with childhood obesity: but is it clinically important? *Int. J. Obes.*, **30**, 171–5.

Hancox, R. J., Milne, B. J., Poulton, R., 2004. Association between child and adolescent television viewing and adult health: a longitudinal birth cohort study. *Lancet*, **364**, 257–62.

Harlow Printing Company, 2007. *Standard Growth Charts*. South Shields, UK: Harlow Printing Company.

Harrell, J. S., McMurray, R. G., Baggett, C. D., Pennell, M. L., Pearce, P. F., Bangdiwala, S. I., 2005. Energy costs of physical activities in children and adolescents. *Med. Sci. Sports Exerc.*, **37**, 329–36.

Harter, S., 1993. Causes and consequences of low self-esteem in children and adolescents. In *The Puzzle of Low Self-Regard*, ed. R. F. Baumeister, pp. 87–116. New York: Plenum Press.

Haslam, D. W., James, W. P. T., 2005. Obesity. *Lancet*, **366**, 1197–209.

Haslam, D., Sattar, N., Lean, M., 2006. Obesity: time to wake up. *Br. Med. J.*, **333**, 640–2.

Hastings, G., Stead, M., McDermott, L., Forsyth, A., MacKintosh, A-M., Rayner, M., Godfrey, C., Caraher, M., Angus, K., 2003. *Review of Research on the Effects of Food Promotion to Children*. London: Foods Standards Agency.

Hayden-Wade, H. A., Stein, R. I., Ghaderi, A., Saelens, B. E., Zabinski, M. F., Wilfley, D. E., 2005. Prevalence, characteristics, and correlates of teasing experiences among overweight children vs. non-overweight peers. *Obes. Res.*, **13**, 1381–92.

Health Survey for England 2004, 2006. *Updating of Trend Tables to Include Childhood Obesity Data*. London: The Stationery Office. Available online at www.ic.nhs.uk/pubs/hsechildobesityupdate

Henderson, R. C., 1992. Tibia vara: a complication of adolescent obesity. *J. Pediatr.*, **121**, 482–6.

Hernandez, B., Gortmaker, S. L., Colditz, G. A., Peterson, K. E., Laird, N. M., Parra-Cabrera, S., 1999. Association of obesity and physical activity, television programs and other forms of video viewing among children in Mexico City. *Int. J. Obes.*, **23**, 845–54.

Hesketh, K., Crawford, D., Salmon, J., 2006. Children's television viewing and objectively measured physical activity: associations with family circumstance. *Int. J. Behav. Nutr. Phys. Act.*, **3**, 36–45.

Hill, C. M., Hogan, A. M., Onugha, N., Harrison, D., Cooper, S., McGrigor, V. J., Dattam A., Kirkham, F. J., 2006. Increased cerebral blood flow velocity in children with mild sleep-disordered breathing: a possible association with abnormal neuropsychological function. *Pediatrics*, **118**, e1100–8.

Hoos, M. B., Kuipers, H., Gerver, W. J., Westerterp, K. R., 2004. Physical activity pattern of children assessed by triaxial accelerometry. *Eur. J. Clin. Nutr.*, **58**, 1425–8.

Hopkinson, Z. E., Sattar, N., Fleming, R., Greer, I. A., 1998. Polycystic ovary syndrome: the metabolic syndrome comes to gynaecology. *Br. Med. J.*, **317**, 329–32.

House of Commons Health Committee, 2004. *Obesity: Third Report of Session 2003/4*. London: HMSO.

Hughes, A. R., Farewell, K., Harris, D., Reilly, J. J., 2007. Quality of life in a clinical sample of obese children. *Int. J. Obes.*, **31**, 39–44.

Huxley, R. R., Neil, H. A., 2004. Does maternal nutrition in pregnancy and birth weight influence levels of CHD risk factors in adult life? *Br. J. Nutr.*, **91**, 459–68.

Huxley, R. R., Neil, A., Collins, R., 2002. Unravelling the fetal origins hypothesis: is there really an inverse association between birthweight and subsequent blood pressure? *Lancet*, **360**, 659–65.

Inge, T. H., Xanthakos, S. A., Zeller, M. H., 2007. Bariatric surgery for pediatric extreme obesity: now or later? *Int. J. Obes.*, **31**, 1–14.

Jackson, L. V., Thalange, N. K., Cole, T. J., 2007. Blood pressure centiles for Great Britain. *Arch. Dis. Child.*, **92**, 298–303.

Jafar, T. H., Chaturvedi, N., Pappas, G., 2006. Prevalence of overweight and obesity and their association with hypertension and diabetes mellitus in an Indo-Asian population. *Can. Med. Assoc. J.*, **175**, 1071–7.

Jain, A., Sherman, S. N., Chamberlin, D. L., Carter, Y., Powers, S. W., Whitaker, RC., 2001. Why don't low-income mothers worry about their preschoolers being overweight? *Pediatrics*, **107**, 1138–46.

James, J., Thomas, P., Cavan, D., Kerr, D., 2004. Preventing childhood obesity by reducing consumption of carbonated drinks: cluster randomized controlled trial. *Br. Med. J.*, **328**, 1237.

Janssen, I., Boyce, W. F., Simpson, K., Pickett, W., 2006. Influence of individual- and area-level measures of socioeconomic status on obesity, unhealthy eating, and physical inactivity in Canadian adolescents. *Am. J. Clin. Nutr.*, **83**, 139–45.

Jebb, S. A., Rennie, K. L., Cole, T. J., 2003. Prevalence and demographic determinants of overweight and obesity among young people in Great Britain. *Int. J. Obes.*, **27**, S9.

Jessup, A., Harrell, J. S., 2005. The metabolic syndrome: look for it in children too. *Clin. Diabetes*, **23**, 26–32.

Kaplowitz, P., 2006. Pubertal development in girls: secular trends. *Curr. Opin. Obstet. Gynecol.*, **18**, 487–91.

Katzmarzyk, P. T., 2004. Waist circumference percentiles for Canadian youth 11–18 y of age. *Eur. J. Clin. Nutr.*, **58**, 1011–15.

Kautianinen, S., Koivusiita, L., Lintonen, T., Virtanen, S. M., Rimpela, A., 2005. Use of information and communication technology and prevalence of overweight and obesity among adolescents. *Int. J. Obes.*, **29**, 925–33.

Kay, J. P., Alemzadeh, R., Langley, G., D'Angelo, L., Smith, P., Holshouser, S., 2001. Beneficial effects of metformin in normoglycemic morbidly obese adolescents. *Metabolism*, **50**, 1457–60.

Keith, S. W., Redden, D. T., Katzmarzyk, P. T., Boggiano, M. M., Hanlon, E. C., Benca, R. M., Ruden, D., Pietrobelli, A., Barger, J. L., Fontaine, K. R., Wang, C., Aronne, L. J., Wright, S. M., Baskin, M., Dhurandhar, N. V., Lijoi, M. C., Grilo,

C. M., DeLuca, M., Westfall, A. O., Allison, D. B., 2006. Putative contributors to the secular increase in obesity: exploring the roads less traveled. *Int. J. Obes.*, **30**, 1585–94.

Kerkar, N., 2004. Non alcoholic steatohepatitits in children. *Pediatr. Transplantation*, **8**, 613–18.

Killen, J. D., Taylor, C. B., Hayward, C., Wilson, D. M., Haydel, K. F., Hammer, L. D., Simmonds, B., Robinson, T. N., Litt, I., Varady, A., 1994. Pursuit of thinness and onset of eating disorder symptoms in a community sample of adolescent girls: a three-year prospective analysis. *Int. J. Eat. Disord.*, **163**, 227–38.

Kinra, S., Nelder, R. P., Lewenden, G. J., 2000. Deprivation and childhood obesity: a cross sectional study of 29 973 children in Plymouth, United Kingdom. *J. Epidemiol. Community Hlth*, **54**, 456–60.

Kleinert, S., 2007. Adolescent health: an opportunity not to be missed. *Lancet*, **369**, 1057–8.

Klesges, R. C., Shelton, M. L., Klesges, L. M.. 1993. Effects of television on metabolic rate: potential implications for childhood obesity. *Pediatrics*, **91**, 281–6.

Kotagal, S., Pianosi, P., 2006. Sleep disorders in children and adolescents. *Br. Med. J.*, **332**, 828–32.

Kral, J. G., 2006. ABC of obesity management: Part III – surgery. *Br. Med. J.*, **333**, 900–3.

Lanigan, J. A., Wells, J. C. K., Lawson, M., Cole, T. J., Lucas, A., 2004. Number of days needed to assess energy and nutrient intake in infants and young children between 6 months and 2 years of age. *Eur. J. Clin. Nutr.*, **58**, 745–50.

Larkin, M., 2003. Can cities be designed to fight obesity? *Lancet*, **362**, 1046–7.

Lawlor, D., Aartin, R. M., Gunell, D., Galobardes, B., Ebrahim, S., Sandhu, J., Ben-Shlomo, Y., McCarron, P., Davey-Smith, G., 2006. Association of body mass index measured in childhood, adolescence and young adulthood with risk of ischemic heart disease and stroke: findings from three historical cohort studies. *Am. J. Clin. Nutr.*, **83**, 767–73.

Laws, R. J., 2004. A new evidence based model for weight management in primary care: the counterweight programme. *J. Hum. Nutr. Diet*, **17**, 191–208.

Lawson, M. L., Kirk, S., Mitchell, T., Chen, M. K., Loux, T. J., Daniels, S. R., Harmon, C. M., Clements, R. H., Garcia, V. F., Inge, T. H., Pediatric Bariatric Study Group, 2006. One-year outcomes of Roux-en-Y gastric bypass for morbidly obese adolescents: a multicenter study from the Pediatric Bariatric Study Group. *J. Pediatr. Surg.*, **41**, 137–43.

Lean, M. E., Han, T. S., Seidell, J. C., 1998. Impairment of health and quality of life in men and women with a large waist. *Lancet*, **351**, 853–6.

Li, H., Stein, A. D., Barnhart, H. X., Ramakrishnan, U., Martorell, R., 2003. Associations between prenatal and postnatal growth and adult body size and composition. *Am. J. Clin. Nutr.*, **77**, 1498–505.

Lissau-Lund-Sørensen, I., Sørensen, T., 1992. Prospective study of the influence of social factors in childhood on risk of overweight in young adulthood. *Int. J. Obes.*, **16**, 169–75.

Lobstein, T., Frelut, M-L., 2003. Prevalence of overweight among children in Europe. *Obes. Rev.*, **4**, 195–200.

Lobstein, T., Baur, L., Uauy, R., 2004. Obesity in children and young people: a crisis in public health. *Obes. Rev.*, **5**, 4–104.

Loder, R. T., Aronsen, D. D., Grenfield, M. L., 1993. The epidemiology of bilateral slipped capital femoral epiphysis: a study of children in Michigan. *J. Bone and Joint Surg.*, **75**, 1141–7.

Lucas, A., Fewtrell, M. S., Cole, T. J., 1999. Fetal origins of adult disease – the hypothesis revisited. *Br. Med. J.*, **319**, 245–9.

Ludwig, D. S., 2007. Clinical update: the low-glycaemic-index diet. *Lancet*, **369**, 890–2.

Lumeng, J. C., Hillman, K. H., 2007. Eating in larger groups increases food consumption. *Arch. Dis. Child.*, **92**, 384–7.

Lustig, R. H., Mietus-Snyder, M. L., Bacchetti, P., Lazar, A. A., Velsquez-Mieyer, P. A., Christensen, M. L., 2006. Insulin dynamics predict body mass index and Z score response to insulin suppression or sensistization pharmacotherapy in obese children. *J. Pediatr.*, **148**, 23–9.

Mackett, R. L., Lucas, L., Paskins, J., Turbin, J., 2003. The health benefits of walking to school. In *Proceedings of the SUSTRANS National Conference on Championing Safe Routes to School: Citizenship in Action.* Available online at www.saferoutesinfo.org

Mamun, A. A., Lawlor, D. A., O'Callaghan, M. J., Williams, G. M., Najman, J. M., 2005. Positive maternal attitude to the family eating together decreases the risk of adolescent overweight. *Obes. Res.*, **13**, 1422–30.

McCarthy, H. D., Jarrett, K. V., Crawley, H. F., 2001. The development of waist circumference percentiles in British children aged 5.0–16.9 y. *Eur. J. Clin. Nutr.*, **55**, 902–7.

McCarthy, H. D., Cole, T. J., Fry, T., Jebb, S. A., Prentice, A. M., 2006. Body fat reference curves for children. *Int. J. Obes.*, **30**, 598–602.

McGarvey, E., Keller, A., Forrester, M., Williams, E., Seward, D., Suttle, D. E., 2004. Feasibility and benefits of a parent-focused preschool child obesity intervention. *Am. J. Publ. Hlth*, **94**, 1490–5.

McMunn, A., Primatesta, P., Bost, L., 2004. *The Health of Young People '95–'97.* London: The Stationery Office.

McPherson, A., 2005. Adolescents in primary care. *Br. Med. J.*, **330**, 465–7.

McQuigg, M., Brown, J., Broom, J., Laws, R. A., Reckless, J. P., Noble, P. A., Kumar, S., McCombie, E. L., Lean, M. E., Lyons, G. F., Frost, G. S., Quinn, M. F., Barth, J. H., Haynes, S. M., Finer, N., Ross, H. M., Hole, D. J., Counterweight Project Team, 2005. Empowering primary care to tackle the obesity epidemic: the Counterweight Programme. *Eur. J. Clin. Nutr.*, **59**, S93–100.

Meier, U., Gressner, A. M., 2004. Endocrine regulation of energy metabolism: review of pathobiochemical and clinical chemical aspects of leptin, ghrelin, adiponectin, and resistin. *Clin. Chem.*, **50**, 1511–25.

Metcalf, B., Voss, L., Jeffery, A., Perkins, J., Wilkin, T., 2004. Physical activity cost of the school run: impact on schoolchildren of being driven to school (EarlyBird 22). *Br. Med. J.*, **329**, 832–3.

Mohammadpour-Ahranjani, B., Rashidi, A., Karandish, M., Eshraghian, M. R., Kalantari, N., 2004. Prevalence of overweight and obesity in adolescent Tehrani students, 2000–2001: an epidemic health problem. *Publ. Hlth Nutr.*, **7**, 645–8.

Morgan, J. B., Williams, P., Foote, K. D., Marriott, L. D., 2006. Do mothers understand healthy eating principles for low-birth-weight infants? *Publ. Hlth Nutr.*, **9**, 700–6.

Murtagh, J., Dixey, R., Rudolf, M., 2006. A qualitative investigation into the levers and barriers to weight loss in children: opinions of obese children. *Arch. Dis. Child.*, **91**, 920–3.

Musaiger, A. O., Al-Ansari, M., Al-Mannai, M., 2000. Anthropometry of adolescent girls in Bahrain, including body fat distribution. *Ann. Hum. Biol.*, **27**, 507–15.

Must, A., Anderson, S. E., 2006. Body mass index in children and adolescents: consideration for population-based approach. *Int. J. Obes.*, **30**, 590–4.

Must, A., Dallal, G. E., Dietz, W. H., 1991. Reference data for obesity: 85th and 95th percentiles of body mass index (wt/ht^2) and triceps skinfold thickness – a correction. *Am. J. Clin. Nutr.*, **54**, 773.

National Audit Office, 2001. *Tackling Obesity*. London: The Stationery Office.

National Institute for Health and Clinical Excellence (NICE), 2006. *Obesity: The Prevention, Identification, Assessment and Management of Overweight and Obesity in Adults and Children.* London: The Stationery Office. Available online at www.nice.org.uk/guidance/CG43

National Obesity Forum, 2007. *Assessment,* Available online at www.nationalobesityforum.org.uk

Nicholls, D., Viner, R., 2005. Eating disorders and weight problems. *Br. Med. J.*, **330**, 950–3.

Northstone, K., Rogers, I., Emmett, P., ALSPAC Team Study, 2002. Drinks consumed by 18-month-old children: are current recommendations being followed? *Eur. J. Clin. Nutr.*, **56**, 236–44.

O'Dea, J. A., 2005. Prevention of child obesity: 'first do not harm'. *Health Educ. Res.*, **20**, 259–65.

Ofcom, 2007. *New Restrictions on the Television Advertising of Food to Children.* London: The Stationery Office. Available online at www.ofcom.org.uk/media/mofaq/bdc/foodadsfaq

Olshansky, S. J., Passaro, D. J., Hershow, R. C., Layden, J., Carnes, B. A., Brody, J., Hayflick, L., Butler, R. N., Allison, D. B., Ludwig, D. S., 2005. A potential decline in life expectancy in the United States in the 21st century. *New Engl. J. Med.*, **352**, 1138–45.

Ong, K. K. L., Ahmed, M. L., Dunger, D. B., 2000. Association between postnatal catch-up growth and obesity in childhood: prospective cohort study. *Br. Med. J.*, **320**, 967–71.

Padwal, R. S., Majumdar, S. R., 2007. Drug treatments for obesity: orlistat, sibutramine and rimonabant. *Lancet*, **369**, 711–77.

Parsons, T. J., Power, C., Manor, O., 2001. Fetal and early life growth and body mass index from birth to early adulthood in the 1958 British cohort: longitudinal study. *Br. Med. J.*, **323**, 1331–5.

Patton, G. C., Viner, R., 2007. Adolescent health: Part 1 – Pubertal transitions in health. *Lancet*, **369**, 1130–9.

Patton, G. C., Selzer, R., Coffey, C., Carlin, J. B., Wolfe, R., 1999. Onset of adolescent eating disorders: population based cohort study over 3 years. *Br. Med. J.*, **318**, 765–8.

Peterson, Y., 2005. Family therapy treatment: working with obese children and their families with small steps and realistic goals. *Acta Paediatr.*, **94**, S42–4.

Petter, L. P., Hourihane, J. O., Rolles, C. J., 1995. Is water out of vogue? A survey of the drinking habits of 2–7 year olds. *Arch. Dis. Child.*, **72**, 137–40.

Phipps, S. A., Burton, P. S., Osberg, L. S., Lethbridge, L. N., 2006. Poverty and the extent of child obesity in Canada, Norway and the United States. *Obes. Rev.*, **7**, 5–12.

Pierce, M. B., Leon, D. A., 2005. Age at menarche and adult BMI in the Aberdeen children of the 1950s cohort study. *Am. J. Clin. Nutr.*, **82**, 733–9.

Pipes, P. L., Holm, V. A., 1980. Feeding children with Down's syndrome. *J. Am. Diet. Assoc.*, **77**, 277–82.

Pinhas-Hamiel, O., Dolan, I. M., Daniels, S. R., Standiford, D., Khoury, P. R., Zeitler, P., 1996. Increased incidence of non-insulin-dependent diabetes mellitus among adolescents. *J. Pediatr.*, **128**, 608–13

Pinhas-Hamiel, O., Singer, S., Pilpel, N., Fradkin, A., Modan, D., Reichman, B., 2006. Health related quality of life among children and adolescents: associations with obesity. *Int. J. Obes.*, **30**, 267–72.

Popkin, B. M., Doak, C. M., 1998. The obesity epidemic is a worldwide phenomenon. *Nutr. Rev.*, **56**, 106–14.

Popkin, B. M., Gordon-Larsen, P., 2004. The nutrition transition: worldwide obesity dynamics and their determinants. *Int. J. Obes.*, **28**, S2–9.

Poskitt, E. M. E., 2002. Home-based management. In *Child and Adolescent Obesity*, ed. W. Burniat, T. Cole, I. Lissau, E. Poskitt, pp. 270–89. Cambridge, UK: Cambridge University Press.

Poskitt, E. M. E., 2005. Tackling childhood obesity: diet, physical activity or lifestyle change? *Acta Paediatr.*, **94**, 396–8.

Poskitt, E. M. E., Cole, T. J., 1977. Do fat babies stay fat? *Br. Med. J.*, **i**, 7–9.

Poskitt, E. M. E., Cole, T. J., 1978. Nature, nurture and childhood overweight. *Br. Med. J.*, **ii**, 603–5.

Poskitt, E. M. E., Clarke, N., Wilkinson, J. L., 1987. Cardiac hypertrophy in obese adolescents. *Int. J. Obes.*, **11**, 87.

Prader–Willi Syndrome Association, 2007. *Home Page.* Available online at http://pwsa.co.uk

Preston, S. H., 2005. Deadweight? The influence of obesity on longevity. *New Engl. J. Med.*, **352**, 1135–7.

Pugliese, M. P., Lifshitz, F., Grad, G., Fort, P., Marks-Katz, M., 1983. Fear of obesity: a cause of short stature and delayed puberty. *New Engl. J. Med.*, **309**, 513–18.

Rauh, J. L., Schumsky, D. A., 1968. Lean and non-lean body mass estimates in urban schoolchildren. In *Human Growth*, ed. D. B. Cheek, pp. 242–52. Philadelphia, PA: Lee & Febiger.

Reilly, J. J., 2006. Diagnostic accuracy of the BMI for age in paediatrics. *Int. J. Obes.*, **30**, 595–7.

Reilly, J. J., Montgomery, C., Jackson, D., MacRitchie, J., Armstrong, J., 2001. Energy intake by multiple pass 24h recall and total energy expenditure: a comparison in a representative sample of 3–4 year olds. *Br. J. Nutr.*, **86**, 601–5.

Reilly, J. J., Armstrong, J., Dorosty, A. R., Emmett, P. M., Ness, A., Rogers, I., Steer, C., Sherriff, A., Avon Longitudinal Study of Parents and Children Study Team, 2005. Early life risk factors for obesity in childhood: cohort study. *Br. Med. J.*, **330**, 1357.

Reinehr, T., 2005. Clinical presentation of type 2 diabetes mellitus in children and adolescents. *Int. J. Obes.*, **29**, S105–10.

Reinehr, T., de Sousa, G., Andler, W., 2005. Longitudinal analyses among overweight, insulin resistance, and cardiovascular risk factors in children. *Obes. Res.*, **13**, 1824–33.

Richards, G. E., Cavalli, A., Meyer, W. J., Price, M. H., Peters, E. H., Stuart, C. A., Smith, E. R., 1985. Obesity, acanthosis nigricans, insulin resistances and hyper-androgenemia: pediatric perspectives and natural history. *J. Pediatr.*, **107**, 893–7.

Riley, D. J., Santiago, T., Edelman, N. H., 1976. Complications of obesity: hypoventilation syndrome in childhood. *Am. J. Dis. Child.*, **130**, 671–4.

Roberts, E. A., 2005. Non-alcoholic fatty liver disease (NAFLD) in children. *Front. Biosci.*, **10**, 2306–18.

Robinson, T. N., Hammer, L. D., Killen, J. D., Kraemer, H. C., Wilson, D. M., Hayward, C., Taylor, C. B., 1993. Does television viewing increase obesity and reduce physical activity? Cross-sectional and longitudinal analyses among adolescent girls. *Pediatrics*, **91**, 273–80.

Rolland-Cachera, M.-F., Deheeger, M., Bellisle, F., Sempé, M., Guilloud-Bataille, M., Patois, E., 1984. Adiposity rebound in children: a simple indicator for predicting obesity. *Am. J. Clin. Nutr.*, **39**, 129–35.

Rolls, B. J., Roe, L. S., Meengs, J. S., 2006. Reductions in portion size and energy density of foods are additive and lead to sustained decreases in energy intake. *Am. J. Clin. Nutr.*, **83**, 11–17.

Romon, M., Duhamel, A., Collinet, N., Weill, J., 2005. Influence of social class on time trends in BMI distribution in 5-year-old French children from 1989 to 1999. *Int. J. Obes.*, **29**, 54–9.

Rosenberg, D. E., Sallis, J. F., Conway, T. L., Cain, K. L., McKenzie, T. L., 2006. Active transportation to school over 2 years in relation to weight status and physical activity. *Obesity*, **14**, 1771–6.

Royal College of General Practitioners/Royal College of Nursing, 2002. *Getting It Right for Teenagers in Your Practice*. London: Royal College of General Practitioners.

Royal College of Paediatrics and Child Health (RCPCH), 2002. *An Approach to Weight Management in Children and Adolescents (2–18 Years) in Primary Care*. London: Royal College of Paediatrics and Child Health.

Royal College of Paediatrics and Child Health, 2003. *Bridging the Gaps: Health Care for Adolescents*. London: Royal College of Paediatrics and Child Health.

Royal College of Physicians, Royal College of Paediatrics and Child Health and the Faculty of Public Health, 2004. *Storing up Problems: The Medical Case for the Slimmer Nation*. London: Royal College of Physicians.

Rudolf, M., Christie, D., McElhone, S., Sahota, P., Dixey, R., Walker, J., Wellings, C., 2006. WATCH IT: a community based programme for obese children and adolescents. *Arch. Dis. Child.*, **91**, 736–9.

Sabin, M. A., Ford, A. L., Holly, J. M., Hunt, L. P., Crowne, E. C., Shield, J. P., 2006. Characterisation of morbidity in a UK, hospital based, obesity clinic. *Arch. Dis. Child.*, **91**, 126–30.

Sacher, P. M., Chadwick, P., Wells, J. C., Williams, J. E., Cole, T. J., Lawson, M. S., 2005. Assessing the acceptability and feasibility of the MEND Programme in a small group of obese 7–11-year-old children. *J. Hum. Nutr. Diet*, **18**, 3–5.

Sahota, P., Rudolf, M. C. J., Dixey, R., Hill, A. J., Barth, J. H., Cade, J., 2001. Evaluation of implementation and effect of primary school based intervention to reduce risk factors for obesity. *Br. Med. J.*, **323**, 1027–9.

Santangelo, A., Peracchi, M., Conte, D., Fraquelli, M., Porrini, M., 1998. Physical state of meal affects gastric emptying, cholecystokinin release and satiety. *Br. J. Nutr.*, **80**, 521–7.

Savoye, M., Berry, D., Dziura, J., Shaw, M., Serrechia, J. B., Barbetta, G., Rose, P., Lavietes, S., Caprio, S., 2005. Anthropometric and psychosocial changes in obese adolescents involved in a weight management program. *J. Am. Dietet. Assoc.*, **105**, 364–70.

Saxena, S., Ambler, G., Cole, T. J., Majeed, A., 2004. Ethnic group differences in overweight and obese children and young people in England: cross sectional survey. *Arch. Dis. Child.*, **89**, 30–6.

Schleimer, K., 1983. Dieting in teenage schoolgirls: a longitudinal prospective study. *Acta Paediatr. Scand.*, **312**, S1–54.

Schrander-Stumpel, C. T., Curfs, L. M., Sastrowijoto, P., Cassidy, S. B., Schrander, J. J., Fryns, J. P., 2004. Prader–Willi syndrome: causes of death in an international series of cases. *Am. J. Med. Genet.*, **124**, 333–8.

Schultz, L. O., Bennett, P. H., Ravussin, E., Kidd, J. R., Kidd, K. K., Esparza, J., Valencia, M. E., 2006. Effects of traditional and western environments on prevalence of type 2 diabetes in Pima Indians in Mexico and the U.S. *Diabetes Care*, **29**, 1866–71.

Schwingshandl, J., Sudi, K., Eibl, B., Wallner, S., Borkenstein, M., 1999. Effect of an individualized training programme during weight reduction on body composition: a randomized trial. *Arch. Dis. Child.*, **81**, 426–8.

Scottish Intercollegiate Guidelines Network (SIGN) Guidelines, 2003. *Management of Obesity in Children and Young People.* Available online at www.sign.ac.uk/guidelines/

Shai, I., Jiang, R., Manson, J. E., Stampfer, M. J., Willett, W. C., Colditz, G. A., Hu, F. B., 2006. Ethnicity, obesity, and risk of type 2 diabetes in women: a 20-year follow-up study. *Diabetes Care*, **29**, 1585–90.

Shukla, A. P., Forsyth, A. A., Anderson, C. M., Marwah, S. M., 1972. Infantile overnutrition in the first year of life: a field study in Dudley, Worcestershire. *Br. Med. J.*, **i**, 507–15.

Silva, A. M., Minderico, C. S., Teixeira, P. J., Pietrobelli, A., Sardinha, L. B., 2006. Body fat measurement in adolescent athletes: multicompartment molecular model comparison. *Eur. J. Clin. Nutr.*, **60**, 955–64.

Singhal, A., Fewtrell, M., Cole, T. J., Lucas, A., 2003. Low nutrient intake and early growth for later insulin resistance in adolescents born preterm. *Lancet*, **361**, 1089–97.

Sørensen, K. H., 1968. Slipped upper femoral epiphysis: clinical study on aetiology. *Acta Orthopaed. Scand.*, **39**, 499–517.

Speiser, P. W., Rudolf, M. C., Anhalt, H., Camacho-Hubner, C., Chiarelli, F., Eliakim, A., Freemark, M., Gruters, A., Hershkovitz, E., Iughetti, L., Krude, H., Latzer, Y., Lustig, R. H., Pescovitz, O. H., Pinhas-Hamiel, O., Rogo, A. D., Shalitin, S., Sultan, C., Stein, D., Vardi, P., Werther, G. A., Zadik, Z., Zuckerman-Levin, N., Hochberg, Z., Obesity Consensus Working Group, 2005. Childhood obesity. *J. Clin. Endocrinol. Metab.*, **90**, 1871–87.

Srinivasan, S. R., Frontini, M. G., Berenson, G. S., 2003. Longitudinal changes in risk variables of insulin resistance syndrome from childhood to young adulthood in offspring of parents with type 2 diabetes: the Bogalusa Heart Study. *Metabolism*, **52**, 443–50.

Srinavasan, S. R., Myers, L., Berenson, G. S., 2006. Changes in metabolic syndrome variables since childhood in prehypertensive and hypertensive subjects: the Bogalusa Heart Study. *Hypertension*, **48**, 21–2.

Stamatakis, E., Primatesta, P., Chinn, S., Rona, R., Falascheti, E., 2005. Overweight and obesity trends from 1974 to 2003 in English children: what is the role of socioeconomic factors? *Arch. Dis. Child.*, **90**, 999–1004.

Stunkard, A. J., Sorensen, T. I., Hanis, C., Teasdale, T. W., Chakraborty, R., Schull, W. J., Schulsinger F. N., 1986. An adoption study of human obesity. *New Engl. J. Med.*, **314**, 193–8.

Stunkard, A. J., Harris, J. R., Pedersen, N. L., McClearn, G. I., 1990. The body mass index of twins who have been reared apart. *New Engl. J. Med.*, **322**, 1483–7.

Sugerman, H. J., Felton, W. L., Sismani, A., 1999. Gastric surgery for pseudotumor cerebri associated with severe obesity. *Ann. Surg.*, **229**, 634–40.

Summerbell, C. D., Waters, E., Edmunds, L., Ashton, V., Campbell, K. J., Kelly, S., 2003. Interventions for treating obesity in children (Cochrane Review). In *The Cochrane Library*, Issue 1. Chichester, UK: John Wiley.

Summerbell, C. D., Waters, E., Edmunds, L. D., Kelly, S., Brown, T., Campbell, K., 2005. Interventions for preventing obesity in children (Cochrane Review). In *The Cochrane Library*, Issue 3. Chichester, UK: John Wiley.

Sustrans, 2007. *Creating the Environment for Active Travel*, Active Travel Information Sheet No. FH09. Bristol, UK: National Cycle Network Centre. Available online at www.sustrans.org/

Swallen, K. C., Reither, E. N., Haas, S. A., Meier, A. M., 2005. Overweight, obesity and health-related quality of life among adolescents: The National Longitudinal Study of Adolescent Health. *Pediatrics*, **115**, 340–7.

Taheri, S., 2006. The link between short sleep duration and obesity: we should recommend more sleep to prevent obesity. *Arch. Dis. Child.*, **91**, 881–4.

Taitz, L. S., 1971. Infant overnutrition among artificially fed infants in the Sheffield region. *Br. Med. J.*, **19**, 315–16.

Tanner, J. M., Whitehouse, R. H., 1975. Revised standards for triceps and subscapular skinfolds in British children. *Arch. Dis. Child.*, **50**, 142–5.

Tate, A. R., Dezetaux, C., Cole, T. J., Millennium Cohort Study Child Health Group, 2006. Is infant growth changing? *Int. J. Obes.*, **30**, 1094–6.

Thompson, G. H., Carter, J. R., 1990. Late onset tibia vara (Blount's disease): current concepts. *Clin. Orthoped.*, **255**, 24–35.

Travers, T., Deem, R., Fox, K. R., Riddoch, C. J., Ness, A. R., Lawlor, D. A., 2006. Improving health through neighbourhood environmental change: are we speaking the same language? A qualitative study of views of different stakeholders. *J. Publ. Hlth*, **28**, 49–55.

Truswell, A. S., Darnton-Hill, I., 1981. Food habits of adolescents. *Nutr. Rev.*, **39**, 73–88.

Turconi, G., Celsa, M., Rezzani, C., Biino, G., Sartirana, M. A., Roggi, C., 2003. Reliability of a dietary questionnaire on food habits, eating behaviour and nutritional knowledge of adolescents. *Eur. J. Clin. Nutr.*, **57**, 753–63.

van den Buick, J., Eggermont, S., 2006. Media use as a reason for meal skipping and fast eating in secondary school children. *J. Hum. Nutr. Diet.*, **19**, 91–100.

Vanhala, M., Vanhala, P., Kupusalo, E., Halonen, P., Takala, J., 1998. Relation between obesity from childhood to adulthood and the metabolic syndrome: population based study. *Br. Med. J.*, **317**, 319–20.

Verhulst, S. L., Schrauwen, N., Haentjens, D., Uys, B., Rooman, R. P., van Gaal, L., de Backer, W. A., Desager, K. N., 2007. Sleep-disordered breathing in overweight and obese children and adolescents: prevalence, characteristics and the role of fat distribution. *Arch. Dis. Child.*, **92**, 224–8.

Vila, G., Zipper, E., Dabbas, M., Bertrand, P. H., Robert, J. J., Ricour, C., Mouren-Siméoni, C., 2004. Mental disorders in obese children and adolescents. *Psychosomatic Med.*, **66**, 387–94.

Viner, R. M., Barker, M., 2005. Young people's health: the need for action. *Br. Med. J.*, **330**, 901–3.

Viner, R. M., Cole, T. J., 2005. Adult socioeconomic, educational, social, and psychological outcomes of childhood obesity: a national birth cohort study. *Br. Med. J.*, **330**, 1354.

Viner, R. M., Segal, T. Y., Lichtarowicz-Krynska, E., Hindmarsh, P., 2005. Prevalence of the insulin resistance syndrome in obesity. *Arch. Dis. Child.*, **90**, 10–14.

Viner, R. M., Haines, M. M., Taylor, S. J. C., Head, J., Booy, R., Stansfeld, S., 2006. Body mass, weight control behaviours, weight perception and emotional well being in a multiethnic sample of early adolescents. *Int. J. Obes.*, **30**, 1514–21.

von Kries, R., Koletzko, B., Sauerwald, T., von Mutius, E., Barnert, D., Grunert, V., van Voss, H., 1999. Breast feeding and obesity: cross sectional study. *Br. Med. J.*, **319**, 147–50.

Wake, M., Hesketh, K., Waters, E., 2003. Television, computer use and body mass index in Australian primary school children. *J. Paediatr. Child Hlth*, **39**, 130–4.

Wang, J., 2006. Standardization of waist circumference reference data. *Am. J. Clin. Nutr.*, **83**, 3–4.

Wang, J., Thornton, J. C., Bari, S., Williamson, B., Gallagher, D., Heymsfield, S. B., Horlick, M., Kotler, D., Laferrere, B., Mayer, L., Pi-Sunyer, F. X., Pierson, R. N. Jr, 2003. Comparisons of waist circumferences measured at four sites. *Am. J. Clin. Nutr.*, **77**, 379–84.

Warburton, D. E., Nicol, C. W., Bredin, S. S., 2006a. Health benefits of physical activity: the evidence. *Can. Med. Assoc. J.*, **174**, 801–9.

Warburton, D. E., Nicol, C. W., Bredin, S. S., 2006b. Prescribing exercise as preventive therapy. *Can. Med. Assoc. J.*, **174**, 961–74.

Wardle, J., Cooke, L., 2005. The impact of obesity on psychological well-being in children. *Best Pract. Res., Clin. Endocrin. Metab.*, **19**, 421–40.

Wardle, J., Volz, C., Goldring, C., 1995. Social variation in attitudes to obesity in children. *Int. J. Obes.*, **19**, 562–9.

Wardle, J., Herrera, M-L., Cooke, L., Gibson, E. L., 2003. Modifying children's food preferences: the effects of exposure and reward on acceptance of an unfamiliar vegetable. *Eur. J. Clin. Nutr.*, **57**, 341–8.

Warren, J. M., Henry, J. K., Simonite, V., 2003. Low glycaemic index breakfasts and reduced food intake in preadolescent children. *Pediatrics*, **112**, 414–19.

Watkins, D., McCarron, P., Murray, L., Cran, G., Boreham, C., Robson, P., McGartland, C., Davey-Smith, G., Savage, M., 2004. Trends in blood pressure over 10 years in adolescents: analyses of cross sectional surveys in the Northern Ireland Young Hearts project. *Br. Med. J.*, **329**, 139–41.

Wells, J. C. K., Fewtrell, M. S., 2006. Measuring body composition. *Arch. Dis. Child.*, **91**, 612–17.

Wells, J. C. K., Fuller, N. J., Wright, A., Fewtrell, M. S., Cole, T. J., 2003. Evaluation of air displacement plethysmography in children aged 5–7 years using a three-compartment model of body composition. *Br. J. Nutr.*, **90**, 699–707.

Westwood, M., Fayter, D., Hartley, S., Rithalia, A., Butler, G., Glasziou, P., Bland, M., Nixon, J., Stirk, L., Rudolf, M., 2007. Childhood obesity: should primary school children be routinely screened? A systematic review and discussion of the evidence. *Arch. Dis. Child.*, **92**, 416–22.

Whincup, P. H., Gilg, J. A., Papacosta, O., Seymour, C., Miller, G. J., Alberti, K. G., Cook, D. G., 2002. Early evidence of ethnic differences in cardiovascular risk: cross sectional comparison of British South Asian and white children. *Br. Med. J.*, **324**, 635.

Whitman, B. Y., Myers, S., Carrel, A., Allen, D., 2002. The behavioural impact of growth hormone treatment for children and adolescents with Prader–Willi syndrome: a 2-year controlled study. *Pediatrics*, **109**, e3.

Widdowson, E. M., 1971. Changes in body proportion and composition during growth. In *Scientific Foundations of Paediatrics*, ed. J. A. Davis, J. Dobbing, pp. 153–64. London: William Heinemann.

Wilcox, P. G., Weiner, D. S., Leighley, B., 1988. Maturation factors in slipped capital femoral epiphysis. *J. Pediatr. Orthoped.*, **8**, 196–200.

Wilkes, M. S., Anderson, 2000. A primary care approach to adolescent health care. *West. J. Med.*, **172**, 177–82.

World Health Organization (WHO), 1983. *Measuring Change in Nutritional Status*. Geneva, Switzerland: World Health Organization.

World Health Organization (WHO), 1998. *Obesity: Preventing and Managing the Global Epidemic*. Report of a WHO Consultation on Obesity, Geneva 3–5 June, 1997. Geneva, Switzerland: World Health Organization.

World Health Organization (WHO), 1999. *Management of Severe Malnutrition: A Manual for Physicians and Other Senior Health Workers*. Geneva, Switzerland: World Health Organization.

World Health Organization (WHO) Expert Committee on Physical Status, 1995. *The Use and Interpretation of Anthropometry.* Geneva, Switzerland: World Health Organization.

Yajnik, C. S., Fall, C. H. D., Coyaji, K. J., Hirve, S. S., Rao, S., Barker, D. J. P., Joglekar, C., Kellingray, S., 2003. Neonatal anthropometry: the thin–fat Indian baby. The Pune Maternal Nutrition Study. *Int. J. Obes.*, **27**, 173–80.

Yitzhak, A., Mizrahi, S., Avinoach, E., 2006. Laparoscopic gastric banding in adolescents. *Obes. Surg.*, **16**, 1318–22.

Yusuf, S., Hawken, S., Ounpuu, S., Bautista, L., Franzosi, M. G., Commerford, P., Lang, C. C., Rumboldt, Z., Onen, C. L., Lisheng, L., Tanomsup, S., Wangai, P. Jr, Razak, F., Sharma, A. M., Anand, S. S. (INTERHEART Study Investigators), 2005. Obesity and the risk of myocardial infarction in 27 000 participants from 52 countries: a case control study. *Lancet*, **366**, 1640–9.

Zaninotto, P., Wardle, H., Stamatakis, E., Mindell, J., Head, J., 2006. *Forecasting Obesity to 2010.* London: The Stationery Office. Available online at www.dh.gov.uk/PublicationsAndStatistics

Index